Mediterranean Diet Cookbook for Beginners

500 Quick and Easy Mouth-watering Recipes that Busy and Novice Can Cook, 2 Weeks Meal Plan Included

By

Wilda Buckley

Table of Content

INTRODUCTION

Mediterranean diet is a specific diet by removing processed foods and/ or high in saturated fats. It's not necessarily about losing weight, but rather a healthy lifestyle choice. It is about ingesting traditional Ingredients consumed by those who live in the Mediterranean basin for a long time. Their diets never changed, so they must be doing something right. This is a diet rich in fruits, vegetables, and fish. Cooking with olive oil is a fundamental ingredient and is an ideal replacement for saturated fats and trans fats. Vegetables and fruits grow well in the heat of the Mediterranean continents, so it's not surprising that the locals devour plenty of them. Studies show that the people who live in these regions live longer and better lives. Changing your own eating habits to one that is proven to be healthy is a good enough reason to begin.

Many studies that have been done on the Mediterranean diet offered promising results.

Heart-healthy diet. Blood pressure tends to drop significantly on the Mediterranean diet; in other words, is a natural way to lower the risk of cardiovascular disease. Researchers have found that the Mediterranean diet can lower your chances of having a stroke and other vascular diseases.

Reduced risk of certain cancers. In general, the Mediterranean diet emphasizes eating plant-based foods and limiting red meat, bad oils, and processed foods. Hence, these eating habits may provide some protection against malignant diseases. People in Mediterranean countries are overall less likely to die from cancer.

Neuroprotective benefits. The Mediterranean diet may improve brain and cogitative functions in older adults (by 15 percent). Clinical trials have shown that those who followed this dietary regimen were less likely to develop Alzheimer's, dementia, or insomnia. A new study has found that antioxidants in the Mediterranean diet plan may protect brain and nerves, cutting the risk of neurological disorders by almost 50 percent.

Weight loss. The Mediterranean diet is the most natural and most delicious way to lose weight and maintain ideal body fat percentage. Low-calorie foods such as fruits, vegetables, yogurt, and fish are widely used in the countries that border the Mediterranean Sea. Natural appetite suppressants include beans, legumes, fat fish, plain dairy products, and high-fiber foods (almost all vegetables, whole grains, apples, avocado, chia seeds). Ginger may control the hunger hormone "ghrelin" too. Consuming a small amount of honey has been shown to reduce appetite. And you will become one step closer to dropping serious pound!

Longevity. Basics of this dietary plan are however vital to longevity and healthy leaving. Other unexpected benefits include reduced risk of developing depression, diabetes management, improved gut health and better mood.

TIPS TO START OFF

Stay Hydrated

Once you've started and are fully immersed in the Mediterranean diet, you might notice that you've started to feel a little bit weak, and a little bit colder, than you're used to. The Mediterranean diet places an emphasis on trying to cut out as much sodium from your diet as possible, which is very healthy for some of us who already have high sodium levels. Sodium, obviously is found in salt, and so we proceed to cut out salt – and then drink enough water to drain every last drop of sodium from our bodies. When it comes to hydration, the biological mechanisms for keeping us saturated and quenched rely on an equal balance of sodium and potassium. Sodium can be found in your interstitial fluid, and potassium can be found inside our cytoplasm – two sides of one wall. When you drink tons of water, sweat a lot at the gym, or both, your sodium leaves your body in your urine and your sweat. Potassium, on the other hand, is only really lost through the urine – and even then, it's rare. This means that our bodies almost constantly need a refill on our sodium levels.

Vitamins and Supplements

Vitamins and minerals can be found in plants and animals, yes, but more often than not fruits and vegetables are much stronger sources. When consume another animal, we are consuming the sum total of all of the energy and nutrition that that animal has also consumed. This might sound like a sweet deal, but the pig you're eating used that energy in his own daily life, and therefore only has a tiny bit left to offer you. Plants, on the other hand, are first-hand sources of things like calcium, vitamin K, and vitamin C, which our bodies require daily doses of.

Meal Preparation and Portion Planning

If you haven't heard of the term "meal prep" before now, it's a beautiful day to learn something that will save you time, stress, and inches on your waistline. Meal prep, short for meal preparation, is a habit that was developed mostly by the body building community in order to accurately track your macronutrients. The basic idea behind meal prep is that each weekend, you manage your free time around cooking and preparing all of your meals for the upcoming week. While most meal preppers do their grocery shopping and cooking on Sundays, to keep their meals the freshest, you can choose to cook on a Saturday if that works better with your schedule. Meal prep each week uses one large grocery list of bulk ingredients to get all the supplies you need to make four dinners and four lunches of your choice. This means that you might have to a bit of mental math quadrupling the serving size, but all you have to do is multiply each ingredient by four. Although you don't have to meal prep more than one meal with four portions each week, if you're already in the kitchen, you most likely have cooking time to work on something else.

Tracking Your Macronutrients

Wouldn't it be nice if you could have a full nutritional label for each of your home-cooked meals, just to make sure that your numbers are adding up in favor of weight loss? Oddly enough, tracking your macronutrients in order to calculate the nutritional value of each of your meals and portions is as easy as stepping on the scale. Not the scale in your bathroom, however. A food scale! If you've never had a good relationship with your weight and numbers, you might suddenly find that they aren't too bad after all. Food scales are used to measure, well, your food, but there's a slick system of online calculators and fitness applications for you smart phone that can take this number and turn it into magic. When you meal prep each week, keep track of your recipes diligently. Remember how you multiplied each of the ingredients on the list by four to create four servings? You're going to want to remember how much of each vegetable, fruit, grain, nut, and fat you cooked with. While you wait for you meal to finish cooking, find a large enough plastic container to fit all of your meal. Make sure it's clean and dry, and use the empty container to zero out your scale.

Counting Calories and Forming a Deficit

When it comes down to the technical science, there is one way and only one way to lose weight: by eating fewer Calories in one day than your body requires to survive. Now, this doesn't mean that you can't lose weight for other reasons – be it water weight, as a result of stress, or simply working out harder. Although counting Calories might not be the most fun way to lose weight, a calorie deficit is the only sure-fire way of guaranteeing that you reap all the weight loss benefits of the Mediterranean diet for your efforts. Scientifically, you already know that the healthy rate of weight loss for the average adult is between one and two pounds per week. Get ready for a little bit more math, but it's nothing you can't handle in the name of a smaller waistline. One pound of fat equals around thirty-five hundred Calories, which means that your caloric deficit needs to account for that number, each week, without making too much a dent on your regular nutrition. For most of us, we're used to eating between fifteen hundred and two thousand Calories per day, which gives you a blessedly simply five hundred calorie deficit per day in order to reach your healthy weight loss goals. If you cut out exactly five hundred Calories each day, you should be able to lose one pound of fat by the end of seven days. Granted, this estimate does take into account thirty minutes of daily exercise, but the results are still about the same when you rely on the scientific facts. If your age, height, weight, and sex predispose you to eat either more or less Calories per day, you might want to consult with your doctor about the healthiest way for you to integrate a caloric deficit into your Mediterranean diet.

Goal Setting to Meet Your Achievements

On the subject of control, there are a few steps and activities that you should go through before you begin your Mediterranean diet just to make sure that you have clear and realistic goals in mind. Sitting down to set goals before embarking on a totally new diet routine will help you stay focused and committed during your Mediterranean diet. While a Mediterranean diet lifestyle certainly isn't as demanding as some of the crazy diet fads you see today, it can be a struggle to focus on eating natural fruits and vegetables that are more "salt of the Earth" foods than we're used to. You already know that when it comes to weight loss, you shouldn't expect to lose more than one to two pounds per week healthily while you're dieting. You are still welcome to set a weight loos goal with time in mind, but when it comes to the Mediterranean diet, you should set your goals for one month in the future.

2-WEEKS MEAL PLAN

DAY	BREAKFAST	LUNCH/DINNER	DESSERT
1.	Avocado Egg Scramble	Delicious Pasta Primavera	Mediterranean Baked Apples
2.	Breakfast Tostadas	Beef with Tomatoes	Mediterranean Diet Cookie Recipe
3.	Parmesan Omelet	Italian Beef	Mediterranean Style Fruit Medley
4.	Menemen	Coriander and Coconut Chicken	Mediterranean Watermelon Salad
5.	Watermelon Pizza	Sage Turkey Mix	Melon Cucumber Smoothie
6.	Ham Muffins	Tasty Greek Rice	Peanut Banana Yogurt Bowl
7.	Baked Oatmeal with Cinnamon	Bulgur salad	Pomegranate and Lychee Sorbet
8.	Creamy Oatmeal with Figs	Lemon Artichokes	Pomegranate Granita with Lychee
9.	Cauliflower Fritters	Turkey and Quinoa Stuffed Peppers	Sweet Tropical Medley Smoothie
10.	Egg Casserole with Paprika	Garlicky Clams	Strawberry Banana Greek Yogurt Parfaits
11.	Avocado Milk Shake	Shrimp, Lemon and Basil Pasta	Summertime Fruit Salad
12.	Banana Quinoa	Quick & Easy Shrimp	Strawberry and Avocado Medley
13.	Morning Pizza with Sprouts	Delicious Pepper Zucchini	Smoothie Bowl with Dragon Fruit
14.	Almond Chia Porridge	Salmon and Watermelon Gazpacho	Roasted Berry and Honey Yogurt Pops

SMOOTHIES & BREAKFASTS RECIPES

1. Avocado Egg Scramble

Preparation time: 8 minutes

Cooking time: 15 minutes

Servings: 4

INGREDIENTS

- 4 eggs, beaten
- 1 white onion, diced
- 1 tablespoon avocado oil
- 1 avocado, finely chopped
- ½ teaspoon chili flakes
- 1 oz Cheddar cheese, shredded
- ½ teaspoon salt
- 1 tablespoon fresh parsley

DIRECTIONS :

1. Pour avocado oil in the skillet and bring it to boil.
2. Then add diced onion and roast it until it is light brown.
3. Meanwhile, mix up together chili flakes, beaten eggs, and salt.
4. Pour the egg mixture over the cooked onion and cook the mixture for 1 minute over the medium heat.
5. After this, scramble the eggs well with the help of the fork or spatula. Cook the eggs until they are solid but soft.
6. After this, add chopped avocado and shredded cheese.
7. Stir the scramble well and transfer in the serving plates.
8. Sprinkle the meal with fresh parsley.

NUTRITION: Calories 236, Fat 20.1, Fiber 4, Carbs 7.4, Protein 8.6

2. Breakfast Tostadas

Preparation time: 15 minutes

Cooking time: 6 minutes

Servings: 6

INGREDIENTS

- ½ white onion, diced
- 1 tomato, chopped
- 1 cucumber, chopped
- 1 tablespoon fresh cilantro, chopped
- ½ jalapeno pepper, chopped
- 1 tablespoon lime juice
- 6 corn tortillas
- 1 tablespoon canola oil
- 2 oz Cheddar cheese, shredded
- ½ cup white beans, canned, drained
- 6 eggs
- ½ teaspoon butter
- ½ teaspoon Sea salt

DIRECTIONS

1. Make Pico de Galo: in the salad bowl combine together diced white onion, tomato, cucumber, fresh cilantro, and jalapeno pepper.
2. Then add lime juice and a ½ tablespoon of canola oil. Mix up the mixture well. Pico de Galo is cooked.
3. After this, preheat the oven to 390F.
4. Line the tray with baking paper.

5. Arrange the corn tortillas on the baking paper and brush with remaining canola oil from both sides.
6. Bake the tortillas for 10 minutes or until they start to be crunchy.
7. Chill the cooked crunchy tortillas well.
8. Meanwhile, toss the butter in the skillet.
9. Crack the eggs in the melted butter and sprinkle them with sea salt.
10. Fry the eggs until the egg whites become white (cooked). Approximately for 3-5 minutes over the medium heat.
11. After this, mash the beans until you get puree texture.
12. Spread the bean puree on the corn tortillas.
13. Add fried eggs.
14. Then top the eggs with Pico de Galo and shredded Cheddar cheese.

NUTRITION: Calories 246, fat 11.1, fiber 4.7, carbs 24.5, protein 13.7

3. Parmesan Omelet

Preparation time: 5 minutes

Cooking time: 10 minutes

Servings: 2

INGREDIENTS

- 1 tablespoon cream cheese
- 2 eggs, beaten
- ¼ teaspoon paprika
- ½ teaspoon dried oregano
- ¼ teaspoon dried dill
- 1 oz Parmesan, grated
- 1 teaspoon coconut oil

DIRECTIONS

1. Mix up together cream cheese with eggs, dried oregano, and dill.
2. Place coconut oil in the skillet and heat it up until it will coat all the skillet.
3. Then pour the egg mixture in the skillet and flatten it.
4. Add grated Parmesan and close the lid.
5. Cook omelet for 10 minutes over the low heat.
6. Then transfer the cooked omelet in the serving plate and sprinkle with paprika.

NUTRITION: Calories 148, fat 11.5, fiber 0.3, carbs 1.4, protein 10.6

4. Menemen

Preparation time: 6 minutes

Cooking time: 15 minutes

Servings: 4

INGREDIENTS

- 2 tomatoes, chopped
- 2 eggs, beaten
- 1 bell pepper, chopped
- 1 teaspoon tomato paste
- ¼ cup of water
- 1 teaspoon butter
- ½ white onion, diced
- ½ teaspoon chili flakes
- 1/3 teaspoon sea salt

DIRECTIONS

1. Put butter in the pan and melt it.
2. Add bell pepper and cook it for 3 minutes over the medium heat. Stir it from time to time.

3. After this, add diced onion and cook it for 2 minutes more.
4. Stir the vegetables and add tomatoes.
5. Cook them for 5 minutes over the medium-low heat.
6. Then add water and tomato paste. Stir well.
7. Add beaten eggs, chili flakes, and sea salt.
8. Stir well and cook menemen for 4 minutes over the medium-low heat.
9. The cooked meal should be half runny.

NUTRITION: Calories 67, fat 3.4, fiber 1.5, carbs 6.4, protein 3.8

5. Watermelon Pizza

Preparation time: 10 minutes

Servings: 2

INGREDIENTS

- 9 oz watermelon slice
- 1 tablespoon Pomegranate sauce
- 2 oz Feta cheese, crumbled
- 1 tablespoon fresh cilantro, chopped

DIRECTIONS

1. Place the watermelon slice in the plate and sprinkle with crumbled Feta cheese.
2. Add fresh cilantro.
3. After this, sprinkle the pizza with Pomegranate juice generously.
4. Cut the pizza into the servings.

NUTRITION: Calories 143, fat 6.2, fiber 0.6, carbs 18.4, protein 5.1

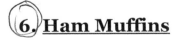 6. Ham Muffins

Preparation time: 10 minutes

Cooking time: 15 minutes

Servings: 4

INGREDIENTS

- 3 oz ham, chopped
- 4 eggs, beaten
- 2 tablespoons coconut flour
- ½ teaspoon dried oregano
- ¼ teaspoon dried cilantro
- Cooking spray

DIRECTIONS

1. Spray the muffin's molds with cooking spray from inside.
2. In the bowl mix up together beaten eggs, coconut flour, dried oregano, cilantro, and ham.
3. When the liquid is homogenous, pour it in the prepared muffin molds.
4. Bake the muffins for 15 minutes at 360F.
5. Chill the cooked meal well and only after this remove from the molds.

NUTRITION: Calories 128, fat 7.2, fiber 2.9, carbs 5.3, protein 10.1

7. Morning Pizza with Sprouts

Preparation time: 15 minutes

Cooking time: 20 minutes

Servings: 6

INGREDIENTS

- ½ cup wheat flour, whole grain
- 2 tablespoons butter, softened

- ¼ teaspoon baking powder
- ¾ teaspoon salt
- 5 oz chicken fillet, boiled
- 2 oz Cheddar cheese, shredded
- 1 teaspoon tomato sauce
- 1 oz bean sprouts

DIRECTIONS

1. Make the pizza crust: mix up together wheat flour, butter, baking powder, and salt. Knead the soft and non-sticky dough. Add more wheat flour if needed.
2. Leave the dough for 10 minutes to chill.
3. Then place the dough on the baking paper. Cover it with the second baking paper sheet.
4. Roll up the dough with the help of the rolling pin to get the round pizza crust.
5. After this, remove the upper baking paper sheet.
6. Transfer the pizza crust in the tray.
7. Spread the crust with tomato sauce.
8. Then shred the chicken fillet and arrange it over the pizza crust.
9. Add shredded Cheddar cheese.
10. Bake pizza for 20 minutes at 355F.
11. Then top the cooked pizza with bean sprouts and slice into the servings.

NUTRITION: Calories 157, fat 8.8, fiber 0.3, carbs 8.4, protein 10.5

8. Banana Quinoa

Preparation time: 10 minutes

Cooking time: 12 minutes

Servings: 4

INGREDIENTS

- 1 cup quinoa
- 2 cup milk
- 1 teaspoon vanilla extract
- 1 teaspoon honey
- 2 bananas, sliced
- ¼ teaspoon ground cinnamon

DIRECTIONS

1. Pour milk in the saucepan and add quinoa.
2. Close the lid and cook it over the medium heat for 12 minutes or until quinoa will absorb all liquid.
3. Then chill the quinoa for 10-15 minutes and place in the serving mason jars.
4. Add honey, vanilla extract, and ground cinnamon.
5. Stir well.
6. Top quinoa with banana and stir it before serving.

NUTRITION: Calories 279, fat 5.3, fiber 4.6, carbs 48.4, protein 10.7

9. Avocado Milk Shake

Preparation time: 10 minutes

Servings: 3

INGREDIENTS

- 1 avocado, peeled, pitted
- 2 tablespoons of liquid honey
- ½ teaspoon vanilla extract
- ½ cup heavy cream
- 1 cup milk
- 1/3 cup ice cubes

DIRECTIONS

1. Chop the avocado and put in the food processor.
2. Add liquid honey, vanilla extract, heavy cream, milk, and ice cubes.
3. Blend the mixture until it smooth.
4. Pour the cooked milkshake in the serving glasses.

NUTRITION: Calories 291, fat 22.1, fiber 4.5, carbs 22, protein 4.4

10. Egg Casserole with Paprika

Preparation time: 10 minutes

Cooking time: 28 minutes

Servings: 4

INGREDIENTS

- 2 eggs, beaten
- 1 red bell pepper, chopped
- 1 chili pepper, chopped
- ½ red onion, diced
- 1 teaspoon canola oil
- ½ teaspoon salt
- 1 teaspoon paprika
- 1 tablespoon fresh cilantro, chopped
- 1 garlic clove, diced
- 1 teaspoon butter, softened
- ¼ teaspoon chili flakes

DIRECTIONS

1. Brush the casserole mold with canola oil and pour beaten eggs inside.
2. After this, toss the butter in the skillet and melt it over the medium heat.
3. Add chili pepper and red bell pepper.
4. After this, add red onion and cook the vegetables for 7-8 minutes over the medium heat. Stir them from time to time.

5. Transfer the vegetables in the casserole mold.
6. Add salt, paprika, cilantro, diced garlic, and chili flakes. Stir gently with the help of a spatula to get a homogenous mixture.
7. Bake the casserole for 20 minutes at 355F in the oven.
8. Then chill the meal well and cut into servings. Transfer the casserole in the serving plates with the help of the spatula.

NUTRITION: Calories 68, fat 4.5, fiber 1, carbs 4.4, protein 3.4

11. Cauliflower Fritters

Preparation time: 10 minutes

Cooking time: 10 minutes

Servings: 2

INGREDIENTS

- 1 cup cauliflower, shredded
- 1 egg, beaten
- 1 tablespoon wheat flour, whole grain
- 1 oz Parmesan, grated
- ½ teaspoon ground black pepper
- 1 tablespoon canola oil

DIRECTIONS

1. In the mixing bowl mix up together shredded cauliflower and egg.
2. Add wheat flour, grated Parmesan, and ground black pepper.
3. Stir the mixture with the help of the fork until it is homogenous and smooth.
4. Pour canola oil in the skillet and bring it to boil.

5. Make the fritters from the cauliflower mixture with the help of the fingertips or use spoon and transfer in the hot oil.
6. Roast the fritters for 4 minutes from each side over the medium-low heat.

NUTRITION: Calories 167, fat 12.3, fiber 1.5, carbs 6.7, protein 8.8

12. Creamy Oatmeal with Figs

Preparation time: 10 minutes

Cooking time: 20 minutes

Servings: 5

INGREDIENTS

- 2 cups oatmeal
- 1 ½ cup milk
- 1 tablespoon butter
- 3 figs, chopped
- 1 tablespoon honey

DIRECTIONS

1. Pour milk in the saucepan.
2. Add oatmeal and close the lid.
3. Cook the oatmeal for 15 minutes over the medium-low heat.
4. Then add chopped figs and honey.
5. Add butter and mix up the oatmeal well.
6. Cook it for 5 minutes more.
7. Close the lid and let the cooked breakfast rest for 10 minutes before serving.

NUTRITION: Calories 222, fat 6, fiber 4.4, carbs 36.5, protein 7.1

13. Baked Oatmeal with Cinnamon

Preparation time: 10 minutes

Cooking time: 25 minutes

Servings: 4

INGREDIENTS

- 1 cup oatmeal
- 1/3 cup milk
- 1 pear, chopped
- 1 teaspoon vanilla extract
- 1 tablespoon Splenda
- 1 teaspoon butter
- ½ teaspoon ground cinnamon
- 1 egg, beaten

DIRECTIONS

1. In the big bowl mix up together oatmeal, milk, egg, vanilla extract, Splenda, and ground cinnamon.
2. Melt butter and add it in the oatmeal mixture.
3. Then add chopped pear and stir it well.
4. Transfer the oatmeal mixture in the casserole mold and flatten gently. Cover it with the foil and secure edges.
5. Bake the oatmeal for 25 minutes at 350F.

NUTRITION: Calories 151, fat 3.9, fiber 3.3, carbs 23.6, protein 4.9

14. Almond Chia Porridge

Preparation time: 10 minutes

Cooking time: 30 minutes

Servings: 4

INGREDIENTS

- 3 cups organic almond milk
- 1/3 cup chia seeds, dried
- 1 teaspoon vanilla extract
- 1 tablespoon honey
- ¼ teaspoon ground cardamom

DIRECTIONS

1. Pour almond milk in the saucepan and bring it to boil.
2. Then chill the almond milk to the room temperature (or appx. For 10-15 minutes).
3. Add vanilla extract, honey, and ground cardamom. Stir well.
4. After this, add chia seeds and stir again.
5. Close the lid and let chia seeds soak the liquid for 20-25 minutes.
6. Transfer the cooked porridge into the serving ramekins.

NUTRITION: Calories 150, fat 7.3, fiber 6.1, carbs 18, protein 3.7

15. Cocoa Oatmeal

Preparation time: 10 minutes

Cooking time: 15 minutes

Servings: 2

INGREDIENTS

- 1 ½ cup oatmeal
- 1 tablespoon cocoa powder
- ½ cup heavy cream
- ¼ cup of water
- 1 teaspoon vanilla extract
- 1 tablespoon butter
- 2 tablespoons Splenda

DIRECTIONS

1. Mix up together oatmeal with cocoa powder and Splenda.
2. Transfer the mixture in the saucepan.
3. Add vanilla extract, water, and heavy cream. Stir it gently with the help of the spatula.
4. Close the lid and cook it for 10-15 minutes over the medium-low heat.
5. Remove the cooked cocoa oatmeal from the heat and add butter. Stir it well.

NUTRITION: Calories 230, fat 10.6, fiber 3.5, carbs 28.1, protein 4.6

16. Cinnamon Roll Oats

Preparation time: 7 minutes

Cooking time: 10 minutes

Servings: 4

INGREDIENTS

- ½ cup rolled oats
- 1 cup milk
- 1 teaspoon vanilla extract
- 1 teaspoon ground cinnamon
- 2 teaspoon honey
- 2 tablespoons Plain yogurt
- 1 teaspoon butter

DIRECTIONS

1. Pour milk in the saucepan and bring it to boil.
2. Add rolled oats and stir well.

3. Close the lid and simmer the oats for 5 minutes over the medium heat. The cooked oats will absorb all milk.
4. Then add butter and stir the oats well.
5. In the separated bowl, whisk together Plain yogurt with honey, cinnamon, and vanilla extract.
6. Transfer the cooked oats in the serving bowls.
7. Top the oats with the yogurt mixture in the shape of the wheel.

NUTRITION: Calories 243, fat 20.2, fiber 1, carbs 2.8, protein 13.3

17. Pumpkin Oatmeal with Spices

Preparation time: 10 minutes

Cooking time: 13 minutes

Servings: 6

INGREDIENTS

- 2 cups oatmeal
- 1 cup of coconut milk
- 1 cup milk
- 1 teaspoon Pumpkin pie spices
- 2 tablespoons pumpkin puree
- 1 tablespoon Honey
- ½ teaspoon butter

DIRECTIONS

1. Pour coconut milk and milk in the saucepan. Add butter and bring the liquid to boil.
2. Add oatmeal, stir well with the help of a spoon and close the lid.
3. Simmer the oatmeal for 7 minutes over the medium heat.

4. Meanwhile, mix up together honey, pumpkin pie spices, and pumpkin puree.
5. When the oatmeal is cooked, add pumpkin puree mixture and stir well.
6. Transfer the cooked breakfast in the serving plates.

NUTRITION: Calories 232, fat 12.5, fiber 3.8, carbs 26.2, protein 5.9

18. Zucchini Oats

Preparation time: 10 minutes

Cooking time: 10 minutes

Servings: 4

INGREDIENTS

- 2 cups rolled oats
- 2 cups of water
- ½ teaspoon salt
- 1 tablespoon butter
- 1 zucchini, grated
- ¼ teaspoon ground ginger

DIRECTIONS

1. Pour water in the saucepan.
2. Add rolled oats, butter, and salt.
3. Stir gently and start to cook the oats for 4 minutes over the high heat.
4. When the mixture starts to boil, add ground ginger and grated zucchini. Stir well.
5. Cook the oats for 5 minutes more over the medium-low heat.

NUTRITION: Calories 189, fat 5.7, fiber 4.7, carbs 29.4, protein 6

19. Breakfast Spanakopita

Preparation time: 15 minutes

Cooking time: 1 hour

Servings: 6

INGREDIENTS

- 2 cups spinach
- 1 white onion, diced
- ½ cup fresh parsley
- 1 teaspoon minced garlic
- 3 oz Feta cheese, crumbled
- 1 teaspoon ground paprika
- 2 eggs, beaten
- 1/3 cup butter, melted
- 2 oz Phyllo dough

DIRECTIONS

1. Separate Phyllo dough into 2 parts.
2. Brush the casserole mold with butter well and place 1 part of Phyllo dough inside.
3. Brush its surface with butter too.
4. Put the spinach and fresh parsley in the blender. Blend it until smooth and transfer in the mixing bowl.
5. Add minced garlic, Feta cheese, ground paprika, eggs, and diced onion. Mix up well.
6. Place the spinach mixture in the casserole mold and flatten it well.
7. Cover the spinach mixture with remaining Phyllo dough and pour remaining butter over it.
8. Bake spanakopita for 1 hour at 350F.
9. Cut it into the servings.

NUTRITION: Calories 190, fat 15.4, fiber 1.1, carbs 8.4, protein 5.4

20. Quinoa Bowl

Preparation time: 10 minutes

Cooking time: 20 minutes

Servings: 4

INGREDIENTS

- 1 sweet potato, peeled, chopped
- 1 tablespoon olive oil
- ½ teaspoon chili flakes
- ½ teaspoon salt
- 1 cup quinoa
- 2 cups of water
- 1 teaspoon butter
- 1 tablespoon fresh cilantro, chopped

DIRECTIONS

1. Line the baking tray with parchment.
2. Arrange the chopped sweet potato in the tray and sprinkle it with chili flakes, salt, and olive oil.
3. Bake the sweet potato for 20 minutes at 355F.
4. Meanwhile, pour water in the saucepan.
5. Add quinoa and cook it over the medium heat for 7 minutes or until quinoa will absorb all liquid.
6. Add butter in the cooked quinoa and stir well.
7. Transfer it in the bowls, add baked sweet potato and chopped cilantro.

NUTRITION: Calories 221, fat 7.1, fiber 3.9, carbs 33.2, protein 6.6

21. Overnight Oats with Nuts

Preparation time: 10 minutes

Cooking time: 8 hours

The super Easy Mediterranean Diet Cookbook for Beginners

Servings: 2

INGREDIENTS

- ½ cup oats
- 2 teaspoons chia seeds, dried
- 1 tablespoon almond, chopped
- ½ teaspoon walnuts, chopped
- 1 cup skim milk
- 2 teaspoons honey
- ½ teaspoon vanilla extract

DIRECTIONS

1. In the big bowl mix up together chia seeds, oats, honey, and vanilla extract.
2. Then add skim milk, walnuts, and almonds. Stir well.
3. Transfer the prepared mixture into the mason jars and close with lids.
4. Put the mason jars in the fridge and leave overnight.
5. Store the meal in the fridge up to 2 days.

NUTRITION: Calories 202, fat 5.4, fiber 4.9, carbs 29.4, protein 8.7

22. Stuffed Figs

Preparation time: 10 minutes

Cooking time: 15 minutes

Servings: 2

INGREDIENTS

- 7 oz fresh figs
- 1 tablespoon cream cheese
- ½ teaspoon walnuts, chopped
- 4 bacon slices
- ¼ teaspoon paprika
- ¼ teaspoon salt
- ½ teaspoon canola oil
- ½ teaspoon honey

DIRECTIONS

1. Make the crosswise cuts in every fig.
2. In the shallow bowl mix up together cream cheese, walnuts, paprika, and salt.
3. Fill the figs with cream cheese mixture and wrap in the bacon.
4. Secure the fruits with toothpicks and sprinkle with honey.
5. Line the baking tray with baking paper.
6. Place the prepared figs in the tray and sprinkle them with olive oil gently.
7. Bake the figs for 15 minutes at 350F.

NUTRITION: Calories 299, fat 19.4, fiber 2.3, carbs 16.7, protein 15.2

23. Poblano Fritatta

Preparation time: 10 minutes

Cooking time: 15 minutes

Servings: 4

INGREDIENTS

- 5 eggs, beaten
- 1 poblano chile, chopped, raw
- 1 oz scallions, chopped
- 1/3 cup heavy cream
- ½ teaspoon butter
- ½ teaspoon salt
- ½ teaspoon chili flakes
- 1 tablespoon fresh cilantro, chopped

DIRECTIONS

1. Mix up together eggs with heavy cream and whisk until homogenous.
2. Add chopped poblano chile, scallions, salt, chili flakes, and fresh cilantro.
3. Toss butter in the skillet and melt it.
4. Add egg mixture and flatten it in the skillet if needed.
5. Close the lid and cook the frittata for 15 minutes over the medium-low heat.
6. When the frittata is cooked, it will be solid.

NUTRITION: Calories 131, fat 10.4, fiber 0.2, carbs 1.3, protein 8.2

24. Mushroom-Egg Casserole

Preparation time: 7 minutes

Cooking time: 25 minutes

Servings: 3

INGREDIENTS

- ½ cup mushrooms, chopped
- ½ yellow onion, diced
- 4 eggs, beaten
- 1 tablespoon coconut flakes
- ½ teaspoon chili pepper
- 1 oz Cheddar cheese, shredded
- 1 teaspoon canola oil

DIRECTIONS

1. Pour canola oil in the skillet and preheat well.
2. Add mushrooms and onion and roast for 5-8 minutes or until the vegetables are light brown.
3. Transfer the cooked vegetables in the casserole mold.
4. Add coconut flakes, chili pepper, and Cheddar cheese.

5. Then add eggs and stir well.
6. Bake the casserole for 15 minutes at 360F.

NUTRITION: Calories 152, fat 11.1, fiber 0.7, carbs 3, protein 10.4

25. Vegetable Breakfast Bowl

Preparation time: 10 minutes

Cooking time: 35 minutes

Servings: 4

INGREDIENTS

- 1 cup sweet potatoes, peeled, chopped
- 1 russet potato, chopped
- 1 red onion, sliced
- 2 bell pepper, trimmed
- ½ teaspoon garlic powder
- ¾ teaspoon onion powder
- 1 tablespoon olive oil
- 1 tablespoon Sriracha sauce
- 1 tablespoon coconut milk

DIRECTIONS

1. Line the baking tray with baking paper.
2. Place the chopped russet potato and sweet potato in the tray.
3. Add onion, bell peppers, and sprinkle the vegetables with olive oil, onion powder, and garlic powder.
4. Mix up the vegetables well with the help of the fingertips and transfer in the preheated to the 360F oven.
5. Bake the vegetables for 45 minutes.
6. Meanwhile, make the sauce: mix up together Sriracha sauce and coconut milk.

7. Transfer the cooked vegetables in the serving plates and sprinkle with Sriracha sauce.

NUTRITION: Calories 213, fat 7.2, fiber 4.8, carbs 34.6, protein 3.6

26. Breakfast Green Smoothie

Preparation time: 7 minutes

Servings: 2

INGREDIENTS

- 2 cups spinach
- 2 cups kale
- 1 cup bok choy
- 1 ½ cup organic almond milk
- 1 tablespoon almonds, chopped
- ½ cup of water

DIRECTIONS

1. Place all ingredients in the blender and blend until you get a smooth mixture.
2. Pour the smoothie in the serving glasses.
3. Add ice cubes if desired.

NUTRITION: Calories 107, fat 3.6, fiber 2.4, carbs 15.5, protein 4.8

27. Simple and Quick Steak

Preparation time: 15 minutes

Cooking time: 10 minutes

Servings: 2

INGREDIENTS

- ½ lb steak, quality - cut

24

- Salt and freshly cracked black pepper

INSTRUCTIONS

1. Switch on the air fryer, set frying basket in it, then set its temperature to 385°F and let preheat.
2. Meanwhile, prepare the steaks, and for this, season steaks with salt and freshly cracked black pepper on both sides.
3. When air fryer has preheated, add prepared steaks in the fryer basket, shut it with lid and cook for 15 minutes.
4. When done, transfer steaks to a dish and then serve immediately.
5. For meal prepping, evenly divide the steaks between two heatproof containers, close them with lid and refrigerate for up to 3 days until ready to serve.
6. When ready to eat, reheat steaks into the microwave until hot and then serve.

NUTRITION: Calories 301, Total Fat 25.1, Total Carbs 0, Protein 19.1g, Sugar 0g, Sodium 65mg

28. Almonds Crusted Rack of Lamb with Rosemary

Preparation time: 10 minutes

Cooking time: 35 minutes

Servings: 2

INGREDIENTS

- 1 garlic clove, minced
- ½ tbsp olive oil
- Salt and freshly cracked black pepper

- ¾ lb rack of lamb
- 1 small organic egg
- 1 tbsp breadcrumbs
- 2 oz almonds, finely chopped
- ½ tbsp fresh rosemary, chopped

INSTRUCTIONS

1. Switch on the oven and set its temperature to 350°F, and let it preheat.
2. Meanwhile, take a baking tray, grease it with oil, and set aside until required.
3. Mix garlic, oil, salt, and freshly cracked black pepper in a bowl and coat the rack of lamb with this garlic, rub on all sides.
4. Crack the egg in a bowl, whisk until blended, and set aside until required.
5. Place breadcrumbs in another dish, add almonds and rosemary and stir until mixed.
6. Dip the seasoned rack of lamb with egg, dredge with the almond mixture until evenly coated on all sides and then place it onto the prepared baking tray.
7. When the oven has preheated, place the rack of lamb in it, and cook for 35 minutes until thoroughly cooked.
8. When done, take out the baking tray, transfer rack of lamb onto a dish, and serve straight away.
9. For meal prep, cut rack of lamb into pieces, evenly divide the lamb between two heatproof containers, close them with lid and refrigerate for up to 3 days until ready to serve.
10. When ready to eat, reheat rack of lamb in the microwave until hot and then serve.

NUTRITION: Calories 471, Total Fat 31.6g, Total Carbs 8.5g, Protein 39g, Sugar 1.5g, Sodium 145mg

29. Cheesy Eggs in Avocado

Preparation time: 20 minutes

Cooking time: 15 minutes

Servings: 2

INGREDIENTS

- 1 medium avocado
- 2 organic eggs
- ¼ cup shredded cheddar cheese
- Salt and freshly cracked black pepper
- 1 tbsp olive oil

INSTRUCTIONS

1. Switch on the oven, then set its temperature to 425°F, and let preheat.
2. Meanwhile, prepare the avocados and for this, cut the avocado in half and remove its pit.
3. Take two muffin tins, grease them with oil, and then add an avocado half into each tin.
4. Crack an egg into each avocado half, season well with salt and freshly cracked black pepper, and then sprinkle cheese on top.
5. When the oven has preheated, place the muffin tins in the oven and bake for 15 minutes until cooked.
6. When done, take out the muffin tins, transfer the avocados baked organic eggs to a dish, and then serve them.

NUTRITION: Calories 210, Total Fat 16.6g, Total Carbs 6.4g, Protein 10.7g, Sugar 2.2g, Sodium 151mg

NUTRITION: Calories 197, Total Fat 13.8g, Total Carbs 4.7g, Protein 14.3g, Sugar 1.9g, Sodium 662mg

30. Bacon, Vegetable and Parmesan Combo

Preparation time: 10 minutes

Cooking time: 25 minutes

Servings: 2

INGREDIENTS

- 2 slices of bacon, thick-cut
- ½ tbsp mayonnaise
- ½ of medium green bell pepper, deseeded, chopped
- 1 scallion, chopped
- ¼ cup grated Parmesan cheese
- 1 tbsp olive oil

INSTRUCTIONS

1. Switch on the oven, then set its temperature to 375°F and let it preheat.
2. Meanwhile, take a baking dish, grease it with oil, and add slices of bacon in it.
3. Spread mayonnaise on top of the bacon, then top with bell peppers and scallions, sprinkle with Parmesan cheese and bake for about 25 minutes until cooked thoroughly.
4. When done, take out the baking dish and serve immediately.
5. For meal prepping, wrap bacon in a plastic sheet and refrigerate for up to 2 days.
6. When ready to eat, reheat bacon in the microwave and then serve.

31. Four-Cheese Zucchini Noodles with Basil Pesto

Preparation time: 10 minutes

Cooking time: 15 minutes

Servings: 2

INGREDIENTS

- 4 cups zucchini noodles
- 4 oz Mascarpone cheese
- 1/8 cup Romano cheese
- 2 tbsp grated parmesan cheese
- ¼ tsp salt
- ½ tsp cracked black pepper
- 2 1/8 tsp ground nutmeg
- 1/8 cup basil pesto
- ½ cup shredded mozzarella cheese
- 1 tbsp olive oil

INSTRUCTIONS

1. Switch on the oven, then set its temperature to 400°F and let it preheat.
2. Meanwhile, place zucchini noodles in a heatproof bowl and microwave at high heat setting for 3 minutes, set aside until required.
3. Take another heatproof bowl, add all cheeses in it, except for mozzarella, season with salt, black pepper and nutmeg, and microwave at high heat setting for 1 minute until cheese has melted.
4. Whisk the cheese mixture, add cooked zucchini noodles in it along

with basil pesto and mozzarella cheese and fold until well mixed.

5. Take a casserole dish, grease it with oil, add zucchini noodles mixture in it, and then bake for 10 minutes until done.

6. Serve straight away.

NUTRITION: Calories 139, Total Fat 9.7g, Total Carbs 3.3, Protein 10.2g, Sodium 419mg, Sugar 0.2g

32. Baked Eggs with Cheddar and Beef

Preparation time: 10 minutes

Cooking time: 20 minutes

Servings: 2

INGREDIENTS

- 3 oz ground beef, cooked
- 2 organic eggs
- 2oz shredded cheddar cheese
- 1 tbsp olive oil

INSTRUCTIONS

1. Switch on the oven, then set its temperature to 390°F and let it preheat.
2. Meanwhile, take a baking dish, grease it with oil, add spread cooked beef in the bottom, then make two holes in it and crack an organic egg into each hole.
3. Sprinkle cheese on top of beef and eggs and bake for 20 minutes until beef has cooked and eggs have set.
4. When done, let baked eggs cool for 5 minutes and then serve straight away.

5. For meal prepping, wrap baked eggs in foil and refrigerate for up to two days.
6. When ready to eat, reheat baked eggs in the microwave and then serve.

NUTRITION: Calories 512, Total Fat 32.8g, Total Carbs 1.4g, Protein 51g, Sugar 1g, Sodium 531mg

33. Heavenly Egg Bake with Blackberry

Preparation time: 10 minutes

Cooking time: 15 minutes

Servings: 4

INGREDIENTS

- Chopped rosemary
- 1 tsp lime zest
- ½ tsp salt
- ¼ tsp vanilla extract, unsweetened
- 1 tsp grated ginger
- 3 tbsp coconut flour
- 1 tbsp unsalted butter
- 5 organic eggs
- 1 tbsp olive oil
- ½ cup fresh blackberries
- Black pepper to taste

INSTRUCTIONS

1. Switch on the oven, then set its temperature to 350°F and let it preheat.
2. Meanwhile, place all the ingredients in a blender, reserving the berries and pulse for 2 to 3 minutes until well blended and smooth.
3. Take four silicon muffin cups, grease them with oil, evenly distribute the

blended batter in the cups, top with black pepper and bake for 15 minutes until cooked through and the top has golden brown.

4. When done, let blueberry egg bake cool in the muffin cups for 5 minutes, then take them out, cool them on a wire rack and then serve.
5. For meal prepping, wrap each egg bake with aluminum foil and freeze for up to 3 days.
6. When ready to eat, reheat blueberry egg bake in the microwave and then serve.

NUTRITION: Calories 144, Total Fat 10g, Total Carbs 2g, Protein 8.5g

34. Protein-Packed Blender Pancakes

Preparation time: 5 minutes

Cooking time: 10 minutes

Servings: 1

INGREDIENTS

- 2 organic eggs
- 1 scoop protein powder
- Salt to taste
- ¼ tsp cinnamon
- 2oz cream cheese, soften
- 1 tsp unsalted butter

INSTRUCTIONS

1. Crack the eggs in a blender, add remaining ingredients except for butter and pulse for 2 minutes until well combined and blended.
2. Take a skillet pan, place it over medium heat, add butter and when it

melts, pour in prepared batter, spread it evenly, and cook for 4 to 5 minutes per side until cooked through and golden brown.

3. Serve straight away.

NUTRITION: Calories 450, Total Fat 29g, Total Carbs 4g, Protein 41g

35. Blueberry and Vanilla Scones

Preparation time: 10 minutes

Cooking time: 10 minutes

Servings: 12

INGREDIENTS

- 1½ cup almond flour
- 3 organic eggs, beaten
- 2 tsp baking powder
- ½ cup stevia
- 2 tsp vanilla extract, unsweetened
- ¾ cup fresh raspberries
- 1 tbsp olive oil

INSTRUCTIONS

1. Switch on the oven, then set its temperature to 375 °F and let it preheat.
2. Take a large bowl, add flour and eggs in it, stir in baking powder, stevia, and vanilla until combined and then fold in berries until mixed.
3. Take a baking dish, grease it with oil, scoop the prepared batter on it with an ice cream scoop and bake for 10 minutes until done.
4. When done, transfer scones on a wire rack, cool them completely, and then serve.

NUTRITION: Calories 133, Total Fat 8g, Total Carbs 4g, Protein 2g

36. Healthy Blueberry and Coconut Smoothie

Preparation time: 5 minutes

Cooking time: 0 minutes

Servings: 2

INGREDIENTS

- 1 cup fresh blueberries
- 1 tsp vanilla extract, unsweetened
- 28 oz coconut milk, unsweetened
- 2 tbsp lemon juice

INSTRUCTIONS

1. Add berries in a blender or food processor, then add remaining ingredients and pulse for 2 minutes until smooth and creamy.
2. Divide the smoothie between two glasses and serve.

NUTRITION: Calories 152, Total Fat 13.1g, Total Carbs 6.9g, Protein 1.5g, Sugar 4.5g, Sodium 1mg

37. Avocado and Eggs Breakfast Tacos

Preparation time: 10 minutes

Cooking time: 13 minutes

Servings: 2

INGREDIENTS

- 4 organic eggs
- 1 tbsp unsalted butter
- 2 low-carb tortillas
- 2 tbsp mayonnaise
- 4 sprigs of cilantro
- ½ of an avocado, sliced
- Salt and freshly cracked black pepper, to taste
- 1 tbsp Tabasco sauce

INSTRUCTIONS

1. Take a bowl, crack eggs in it and whisk well until smooth.
2. Take a skillet pan, place it over medium heat, add butter and when it melts, pour in eggs, spread them evenly in the pan and cook for 4 to 5 minutes until done.
3. When done, transfer eggs to a plate and set aside until required.
4. Add tortillas into the pan, cook for 2 to 3 minutes per side until warm through, and then transfer them onto a plate.
5. Assemble tacos and for this, spread mayonnaise on the side of each tortilla, then distribute cooked eggs, and top with cilantro and sliced avocado.
6. Season with salt and black pepper, drizzle with tabasco sauce, and roll up the tortillas.
7. Serve straight away or store in the refrigerator for up to 2 days until ready to eat.

NUTRITION: Calories 289, Total Fat 27g, Total Carbs 6g, Protein 7g

38. Delicious Frittata with Brie and Bacon

Preparation time: 10 minutes

Cooking time: 20 minutes

Servings: 2

INGREDIENTS

- 4 slices of bacon
- 4 organic eggs, beaten
- ½ cup heavy cream
- Salt and freshly cracked black pepper, to taste
- 4 oz brie, diced
- 1 ½ cup of water
- 1 tbsp olive oil

INSTRUCTIONS

1. Switch on the instant pot, insert its inner pot, press the 'sauté' button, and when hot, add bacon slices and cook for 5 to 7 minutes until crispy.
2. Then transfer bacon to a plate lined with paper towels to drain grease and set aside until required.
3. Crack eggs in a bowl, add cream, season with salt and black pepper and whisk until combined.
4. Chop the cooked bacon, add to the eggs along with brie and stir until mixed.
5. Take a baking dish, grease it with oil, pour in the egg mixture, and spread evenly.
6. Carefully pour water into the instant pot, insert a trivet stand, place baking dish on it, shut with lid, then press the 'manual' button and cook the frittata for 20 minutes at high-pressure setting.
7. When the timer beeps, press the 'cancel' button, allow pressure to release naturally until pressure valve drops, then open the lid and take out the baking dish.
8. Wipe clean moisture on top of the frittata with a paper towel and let it cool completely.
9. For meal prep, cut frittata into six slices, then place each slice in a plastic bag or airtight container and store in the refrigerator for up to three days or store in the freezer until ready to eat.

NUTRITION: Calories 210, Total Fat 19g, Saturated Fat 8g, Total Carbs 3g, Protein 13g, Fiber 0g

39. Awesome Coffee with Butter

Preparation time: 5 minutes

Cooking time: 5 minutes

Servings: 1

INGREDIENTS

- 1 cup of water
- 1 tbsp coconut oil
- 1 tbsp unsalted butter
- 2 tbsp coffee

INSTRUCTIONS

1. Take a small pan, place it over medium heat, pour in water, and bring to boil.
2. Then add remaining ingredients, stir well, and cook until butter and oil have melted.
3. Remove pan from heat, pass the coffee through a strainer, and serve immediately.

NUTRITION: Calories 230, Total Fat 25g, Total Carbs 0g, Protein 0g

40. Buttered Thyme Scallops

Preparation time: 10 minutes

Cooking time: 5 minutes

Servings: 2

INGREDIENTS

- ¾ lb sea scallops
- ½ tbsp fresh minced thyme
- Salt and freshly cracked black pepper, to taste
- 1 tbsp unsalted butter, melted
- 1 tbsp olive oil

INSTRUCTIONS

1. Switch on the oven, then set its temperature to 390°F and let it preheat.
2. Take a large bowl, add all the ingredients in it and toss until well coated.
3. Take a baking dish, grease it with oil, add prepared scallop mixture in it and bake for 5 minutes until thoroughly cooked.
4. When done, take out the baking dish, then scallops cool for 5 minutes and then serve.
5. For meal prepping, transfer scallops into an airtight container and store in the refrigerator for up to two days.
6. When ready to eat, reheat scallops in the microwave until hot and then serve.

NUTRITION: Calories 202, Total Fat 7.1g, Total Carbs 4.4g, Protein 28.7g, Sugar 0g, Sodium 315mg

41. Cheesy Caprese Style Portobellos Mushrooms

Preparation time: 5 minutes

Cooking time: 15 minutes

Servings: 2

INGREDIENTS

- 2 large caps of Portobello mushroom, gills removed
- 4 tomatoes, halved
- Salt and freshly cracked black pepper, to taste
- ¼ cup fresh basil
- 4 tbsp olive oil
- ¼ cup shredded Mozzarella cheese

INSTRUCTIONS

1. Switch on the oven, then set i temperature to 400°F and let preheat.
2. Meanwhile, prepare mushrooms, for this, brush them with olive oil set aside until required.
3. Place tomatoes in a bowl, season salt and black pepper, add drizzle with oil and toss until mix
4. Distribute cheese evenly in the of each mushroom cap and t' with prepared tomato mixture.
5. Take a baking sheet, line aluminum foil, place mushrooms on it and bak minutes until thoroughly coo
6. Serve straight away.

NUTRITION: Calories 315, Total Fat 29.2g, Total Carbs 14.2g, Protein 4.7g, Sugar 10.4g, Sodium 55mg

42. Persimmon Toast with Cream Cheese

Preparation time: 5 minutes

Cooking time: 3 minutes

Servings: 2

INGREDIENTS

- 2 slices whole-grain bread
- 1 persimmon
- 2 teaspoons cream cheese
- 1 teaspoon honey

~RECTIONS

Toast the bread with the help of the toaster. You should get light brown ~read slices.

~ter this, slice persimmon.

~ead the cream cheese on the ~ted bread and top it with sliced ~mmon.

~prinkle very toast with honey.

~alories 107, fat 2.2, fiber 1.9, ~ in 4

~d Eggs

it with ~ns
~repared
~ for 15
~ed.

- Salt and black pepper, to taste

DIRECTIONS

1. Combine together eggs, salt and black pepper in a bowl and keep aside.
2. Heat butter in a pan over medium-low heat and slowly add the whisked eggs.
3. Stir the eggs continuously in the pan with the help of a fork for about 4 minutes.
4. Dish out in a plate and serve immediately.
5. You can refrigerate this scramble for about 2 days for meal prepping and reuse by heating it in microwave oven.

NUTRITION:Calories: 151 , **Fat:** 11.6g **Carbohydrates:** 0.7g **Protein:** 11.1g **Sodium:** 144mg **Sugar:** 0.7g

44. Bacon Veggies Combo

Servings: 2

Preparation time: 35 mins

INGREDIENTS

- ½ green bell pepper, seeded and chopped
- 2 bacon slices
- ¼ cup Parmesan Cheese
- ½ tablespoon mayonnaise
- 1 scallion, chopped

DIRECTIONS

1. Preheat the oven to 375 degrees F and grease a baking dish.
2. Place bacon slices on the baking dish and top with mayonnaise, bell peppers, scallions and Parmesan Cheese.

3. Transfer in the oven and bake for about 25 minutes.
4. Dish out to serve immediately or refrigerate for about 2 days wrapped in a plastic sheet for meal prepping.

NUTRITION:Calories: 197 **Fat:** 13.8g **Carbohydrates:** 4.7g **Protein:** 14.3g **Sugar:** 1.9g **Sodium:** 662mg

45. Tofu with Mushrooms

Servings: 2

Preparation time: 25 mins

INGREDIENTS

- 1 cup fresh mushrooms, chopped finely
- 1 block tofu, pressed and cubed into 1-inch pieces
- 4 tablespoons butter
- Salt and black pepper, to taste
- 4 tablespoons Parmesan cheese, shredded

DIRECTIONS

1. Season the tofu with salt and black pepper.
2. Put butter and seasoned tofu in a pan and cook for about 5 minutes.
3. Add mushrooms and Parmesan cheese and cook for another 5 minutes, stirring occasionally.
4. Dish out and serve immediately or refrigerate for about 3 days wrapped in a foil for meal prepping and microwave it to serve again.

NUTRITION:Calories: 423 **Fat:** 37g **Carbohydrates:** 4g **Protein:** 23.1g **Sugar:** 0.9g **Sodium:** 691mg

46. Ham Spinach Ballet

Servings: 2

Preparation time: 40 mins

INGREDIENTS

- 4 teaspoons cream
- ¾ pound fresh baby spinach
- 7-ounce ham, sliced
- Salt and black pepper, to taste
- 1 tablespoon unsalted butter, melted

DIRECTIONS

1. Preheat the oven to 360 degrees F. and grease 2 ramekins with butter.
2. Put butter and spinach in a skillet and cook for about 3 minutes.
3. Add cooked spinach in the ramekins and top with ham slices, cream, salt and black pepper.
4. Bake for about 25 minutes and dish out to serve hot.
5. For meal prepping, you can refrigerate this ham spinach ballet for about 3 days wrapped in a foil.

NUTRITION:Calories: 188 **Fat:** 12.5g **Carbohydrates:** 4.9g **Protein:** 14.6g **Sugar:** 0.3g **Sodium:** 1098mg

47. Creamy Parsley Soufflé

Servings: 2

Preparation time: 25 mins

The super Easy Mediterranean Diet Cookbook for Beginners

INGREDIENTS

- 2 fresh red chili peppers, chopped
- Salt, to taste
- 4 eggs
- 4 tablespoons light cream
- 2 tablespoons fresh parsley, chopped

DIRECTIONS

1. Preheat the oven to 375 degrees F and grease 2 soufflé dishes.
2. Combine all the ingredients in a bowl and mix well.
3. Put the mixture into prepared soufflé dishes and transfer in the oven.
4. Cook for about 6 minutes and dish out to serve immediately.
5. For meal prepping, you can refrigerate this creamy parsley soufflé in the ramekins covered in a foil for about 2-3 days.

NUTRITION:Calories: 108 **Fat:** 9g Carbohydrates: 1.1g Protein: 6g Sugar: 0.5g Sodium: 146mg

48. **Vegetarian Three Cheese Quiche Stuffed Peppers**

Servings: 2

Preparation time: 50 mins

INGREDIENTS

- 2 large eggs
- ¼ cup mozzarella, shredded
- 1 medium bell peppers, sliced in half and seeds removed
- ¼ cup ricotta cheese
- ¼ cup grated Parmesan cheese
- ½ teaspoon garlic powder

- 1/8 cup baby spinach leaves
- ¼ teaspoon dried parsley
- 1 tablespoon Parmesan cheese, to garnish

DIRECTIONS

1. Preheat oven to 375 degrees F.
2. Blend all the cheeses, eggs, garlic powder and parsley in a food processor and process until smooth.
3. Pour the cheese mixture into each sliced bell pepper and top with spinach leaves.
4. Stir with a fork, pushing them under the cheese mixture and cover with foil.
5. Bake for about 40 minutes and sprinkle with Parmesan cheese.
6. Broil for about 5 minutes and dish out to serve.

NUTRITION: Calories: 157 **Carbs:** 7.3g **Fats:** 9g **Proteins:** 12.7g **Sodium:** 166mg **Sugar:** 3.7g

49. **Spinach Artichoke Egg Casserole**

Servings: 2

Preparation time: 45 mins

INGREDIENTS

- 1/8 cup milk
- 2.5-ounce frozen chopped spinach, thawed and drained well
- 1/8 cup parmesan cheese
- 1/8 cup onions, shaved
- ¼ teaspoon salt
- ¼ teaspoon crushed red pepper
- 4 large eggs
- 3.5-ounce artichoke hearts, drained

- ¼ cup white cheddar, shredded
- 1/8 cup ricotta cheese
- ½ garlic clove, minced
- ¼ teaspoon dried thyme

DIRECTIONS

1. Preheat the oven to 350 degrees F and grease a baking dish with non-stick cooking spray.
2. Whisk eggs and milk together and add artichoke hearts and spinach.
3. Mix well and stir in rest of the ingredients, withholding the ricotta cheese.
4. Pour the mixture into the baking dish and top evenly with ricotta cheese.
5. Transfer in the oven and bake for about 30 minutes.
6. Dish out and serve warm.

NUTRITION: **Calories:** 228 Carbs: 10.1g Fats: 13.3g Proteins: 19.1g Sodium: 571mg Sugar: 2.5g

50. **Avocado Baked Eggs**

Servings: 2

Preparation time: 25 mins

INGREDIENTS

- 2 eggs
- 1 medium sized avocado, halved and pit removed
- ¼ cup cheddar cheese, shredded
- Kosher salt and black pepper, to taste

DIRECTIONS

1. Preheat oven to 425 degrees and grease a muffin pan.

2. Crack open an egg into each half of the avocado and season with salt and black pepper.
3. Top with cheddar cheese and transfer the muffin pan in the oven.
4. Bake for about 15 minutes and dish out to serve.

NUTRITION: **Calories:** 210 Carbs: 6.4g Fats: 16.6g Proteins: 10.7g Sodium: 151mg Sugar: 2.2g

51. **Cinnamon Faux-St Crunch Cereal**

Servings: 2

Preparation time: 35 mins

INGREDIENTS

- ¼ cup hulled hemp seeds
- ½ tablespoon coconut oil
- ¼ cup milled flax seed
- 1 tablespoon ground cinnamon
- ¼ cup apple juice

DIRECTIONS

1. Preheat the oven to 300 degrees F and line a cookie sheet with parchment paper.
2. Put hemp seeds, flax seed and ground cinnamon in a food processor.
3. Add coconut oil and apple juice and blend until smooth.
4. Pour the mixture on the cookie sheet and transfer in the oven.
5. Bake for about 15 minutes and lower the temperature of the oven to 250 degrees F.
6. Bake for another 10 minutes and dish out from the oven, turning it off.

7. Cut into small squares and place in the turned off oven.
8. Place the cereal in the oven for 1 hour until it is crisp.
9. Dish out and serve with unsweetened almond milk.

NUTRITION: **Calories:** 225 Carbs: 9.2g Fats: 18.5g Proteins: 9.8g Sodium: 1mg Sugar: 1.6g

52. Quick Keto McMuffins

Servings: 2

Preparation time: 15 mins

INGREDIENTS

Muffins:

- ¼ cup flaxmeal
- ¼ cup almond flour
- ¼ teaspoon baking soda
- 1 large egg, free-range or organic
- 2 tablespoons water
- 1 pinch salt
- 2 tablespoons heavy whipping cream
- ¼ cup cheddar cheese, grated

Filling:

- 1 tablespoon ghee
- 2 slices cheddar cheese
- Salt and black pepper, to taste
- 2 large eggs
- 1 tablespoon butter
- 1 teaspoon Dijon mustard

DIRECTIONS
For Muffins:

1. Mix together all the dry ingredients for muffins in a small bowl and add egg, cream, cheese and water.

2. Combine well and pour in 2 single-serving ramekins.
3. Microwave on high for about 90 seconds.

For Filling:

4. Fry the eggs on ghee and season with salt and black pepper.
5. Cut the muffins in half and spread butter on the inside of each half.
6. Top each buttered half with cheese slices, eggs and Dijon mustard.
7. Serve immediately.

NUTRITION: **Calories:** 299 Carbs: 8.8g Fats: 24.3g Proteins: 13g Sodium: 376mg Sugar: 0.4g

53. Keto Egg Fast Snickerdoodle Crepes

Servings: 2

Preparation time: 15 mins

INGREDIENTS

For the crepes:

- 5 oz cream cheese, softened
- 6 eggs
- 1 teaspoon cinnamon
- Butter, for frying
- 1 tablespoon Swerve

For the filling:

- 2 tablespoons granulated Swerve
- 8 tablespoons butter, softened
- 1 tablespoon cinnamon

DIRECTIONS

1. For the crepes: Put all the ingredients together in a blender except the butter and process until smooth.
2. Heat butter on medium heat in a non-stick pan and pour some batter in the pan.
3. Cook for about 2 minutes, then flip and cook for 2 more minutes.
4. Repeat with the remaining mixture.
5. Mix Swerve, butter and cinnamon in a small bowl until combined.
6. Spread this mixture onto the centre of the crepe and serve rolled up.

NUTRITION: Calories: 543 **Carbs:** 8g **Fats:** 51.6g **Proteins:** 15.7g **Sodium:** 455mg **Sugar:** 0.9g

54. Cauliflower Hash Brown Breakfast Bowl

Servings: 2

Preparation time: 30 mins

INGREDIENTS

- 1 tablespoon lemon juice
- 1 egg
- 1 avocado
- 1 teaspoon garlic powder
- 2 tablespoons extra virgin olive oil
- 2 oz mushrooms, sliced
- ½ green onion, chopped
- ¼ cup salsa
- ¾ cup cauliflower rice
- ½ small handful baby spinach
- Salt and black pepper, to taste

DIRECTIONS

1. Mash together avocado, lemon juice, garlic powder, salt and black pepper in a small bowl.
2. Whisk eggs, salt and black pepper in a bowl and keep aside.
3. Heat half of olive oil over medium heat in a skillet and add mushrooms.
4. Sauté for about 3 minutes and season with garlic powder, salt, and pepper.
5. Sauté for about 2 minutes and dish out in a bowl.
6. Add rest of the olive oil and add cauliflower, garlic powder, salt and pepper.
7. Sauté for about 5 minutes and dish out.
8. Return the mushrooms to the skillet and add green onions and baby spinach.
9. Sauté for about 30 seconds and add whisked eggs.
10. Sauté for about 1 minute and scoop on the sautéed cauliflower hash browns.
11. Top with salsa and mashed avocado and serve.

NUTRITION: Calories: 400 **Carbs:** 15.8g **Fats:** 36.7g **Proteins:** 8g **Sodium:** 288mg **Sugar:** 4.2g

55. Cheesy Thyme Waffles

Servings: 2

Preparation time: 15 mins

INGREDIENTS

- ½ cup mozzarella cheese, finely shredded
- ¼ cup Parmesan cheese

- ¼ large head cauliflower
- ½ cup collard greens
- 1 large egg
- 1 stalk green onion
- ½ tablespoon olive oil
- ½ teaspoon garlic powder
- ¼ teaspoon salt
- ½ tablespoon sesame seed
- 1 teaspoon fresh thyme, chopped
- ¼ teaspoon ground black pepper

DIRECTIONS

1. Put cauliflower, collard greens, spring onion and thyme in a food processor and pulse until smooth.
2. Dish out the mixture in a bowl and stir in rest of the ingredients.
3. Heat a waffle iron and transfer the mixture evenly over the griddle.
4. Cook until a waffle is formed and dish out in a serving platter.

NUTRITION: Calories: 144 Carbs: 8.5g Fats: 9.4g Proteins: 9.3g Sodium: 435mg Sugar: 3g

56. Baked Eggs and Asparagus with Parmesan

Servings: 2

Preparation time: 30 mins

INGREDIENTS

- 4 eggs
- 8 thick asparagus spears, cut into bite-sized pieces
- 2 teaspoons olive oil
- 2 tablespoons Parmesan cheese
- Salt and black pepper, to taste

DIRECTIONS

1. Preheat the oven to 400 degrees F and grease two gratin dishes with olive oil.
2. Put half the asparagus into each gratin dish and place in the oven.
3. Roast for about 10 minutes and dish out the gratin dishes.
4. Crack eggs over the asparagus and transfer into the oven.
5. Bake for about 5 minutes and dish out the gratin dishes.
6. Sprinkle with Parmesan cheese and put the dishes back in the oven.
7. Bake for another 3 minutes and dish out to serve hot.

NUTRITION: Calories: 336 Carbs: 13.7g Fats: 19.4g Proteins: 28.1g Sodium: 2103mg Sugar: 4.7g

57. Low Carb Green Smoothie

Servings: 2

Preparation time: 15 mins

INGREDIENTS

- 1/3 cup romaine lettuce
- 1/3 tablespoon fresh ginger, peeled and chopped
- 1½ cups filtered water
- 1/8 cup fresh pineapple, chopped
- ¾ tablespoon fresh parsley
- 1/3 cup raw cucumber, peeled and sliced
- ¼ Hass avocado
- ¼ cup kiwi fruit, peeled and chopped
- 1/3 tablespoon Swerve

DIRECTIONS

1. Put all the ingredients in a blender and blend until smooth.
2. Pour into 2 serving glasses and serve chilled.

NUTRITION: **Calories:** 108 Carbs: 7.8g Fats: 8.9g Proteins: 1.6g Sodium: 4mg Sugar: 2.2g

SALADS

58. Lentil Salmon Salad

Servings 4

Preparation and Cooking Time 25 minutes

INGREDIENTS

- Vegetable stock - 2 cups
- Green lentils - 1, rinsed
- Red onion - 1, chopped
- Parsley - 1 2 cup, chopped
- Smoked salmon - 4 oz., shredded
- Cilantro - 2 tbsp., chopped
- Red pepper - 1, chopped
- Lemon - 1, juiced
- Salt and pepper - to taste

DIRECTIONS

1. Cook vegetable stock and lentils in a sauce pan for 15 to 20 minutes, on low heat. Ensure all liquid has been absorbed and then remove from heat.
2. Pour into a salad bowl and top with red pepper, parsley, cilantro and salt and pepper (to suit your taste) and mix.
3. Mix in lemon juice and shredded salmon.
4. This salad should be served fresh.

59. Peppy Pepper Tomato Salad

Servings 4

Preparation Time 20 minutes

INGREDIENTS

- Yellow bell pepper - 1, cored and diced
- Cucumbers - 4, diced
- Red onion - 1, chopped
- Balsamic vinegar – 1 tbsp.
- Extra virgin olive oil – 2 tbsp.
- Tomatoes - 4, diced
- Red bell peppers - 2, cored and diced
- Chili flakes - 1 pinch
- Salt and pepper - to taste

DIRECTIONS

1. Mix all above Ingredients in a salad bowl, except salt and pepper.
2. Season with salt and pepper to suit your taste and mix well.
3. Eat while fresh.

60. Bulgur Salad

Servings 4

Preparation and Cooking Time 30 minutes

INGREDIENTS

- Vegetable stock - 2 cups
- Bulgur - 2 3 cup
- Garlic clove - 1, minced
- Cherry tomatoes - 1 cup, halved
- Almonds - 2 tbsp., sliced
- Dates - 1 4 cup, pitted and chopped
- Lemon juice - 1 tbsp.
- Baby spinach - 8 oz.
- Cucumber - 1, diced
- Balsamic vinegar - 1 tbsp.
- Salt and pepper - to taste

- Mixed seeds - 2 tbsp.

DIRECTIONS

1. Pour stock into sauce pan and heat until hot, then stir in bulgur and cook until bulgur has absorbed all stock.
2. Put in salad bowl and add remaining Ingredients:, stir well.
3. Add salt and pepper to suit your taste.
4. Serve and eat immediately.

61. Tasty Tuna Salad

Servings 4

Preparation Time 15 minutes

INGREDIENTS

- Green olives - 1 4 cup, sliced
- Tuna in water - 1 can, drained
- Pine nuts - 2 tbsp.
- Artichoke hearts – 1 jar, drained and chopped
- Extra virgin olive oil - 2 tbsp.
- Lemon – 1, juiced
- Arugula - 2 leaves
- Dijon mustard - 1 tbsp.
- Salt and pepper - to taste

DIRECTIONS

1. Mix mustard, oil and lemon juice in a bowl to make a dressing. Combine the artichoke hearts, tuna, green olives, arugula and pine nuts in a salad bowl.
2. In a separate salad bowl, mix tuna, arugula, pine nuts, artichoke hearts and tuna.

3. Pour dressing mix onto salad and serve fresh.

62. Sweet and Sour Spinach Salad

Servings 4

Preparation Time 15 minutes

INGREDIENTS

- Red onions - 2, sliced
- Baby spinach leaves - 4
- Sesame oil - 1 2 tsp.
- Apple cider vinegar - 2 tbsp.
- Honey - 1 tsp.
- Sesame seeds - 2 tbsp.
- Salt and pepper - to taste

DIRECTIONS

1. Mix together honey, sesame oil, vinegar and sesame seeds in a small bowl to make a dressing. Add in salt and pepper to suit your taste.
2. Add red onions and spinach together in a salad bowl.
3. Pour dressing over the salad and serve while cool and fresh.

63. Easy Eggplant Salad

Servings 4

Preparation Time 30 minutes

INGREDIENTS

- Salt and pepper - to taste
- Eggplant - 2, sliced
- Smoked paprika - 1 tsp.
- Extra virgin olive oil - 2 tbsp.
- Garlic cloves - 2, minced

- Mixed greens - 2 cups
- Sherry vinegar - 2 tbsp.

DIRECTIONS

1. Mix together garlic, paprika and oil in a small bowl.
2. Place eggplant on a plate and sprinkle with salt and pepper to suit your taste. Next, brush oil mixture onto the eggplant.
3. Cook eggplant on a medium heated grill pan until brown on both sides. Once cooked, put eggplant into a salad bowl.
4. Top with greens and vinegar and greens, serve and eat.

64. **Sweetest Sweet Potato Salad**

Servings 4

Preparation and Cooking Time 30 minutes

INGREDIENTS

- Honey - 2 tbsp.
- Sumac spice - 1 tsp.
- Sweet potato - 2, finely sliced
- Extra virgin olive oil - 3 tbsp.
- Dried mint - 1 tsp.
- Balsamic vinegar – 1 tbsp.
- Salt and pepper - to taste
- Pomegranate - 1, seeded
- Mixed greens - 3 cups

DIRECTIONS

1. Place sweet potato slices on a plate and add sumac, mint, salt and pepper on both sides. Next, drizzle oil and honey over both sides.

2. Add oil to a grill pan and heat. Grill sweet potatoes on medium heat until brown on both sides.
3. Put sweet potatoes in a salad bowl and top with pomegranate and mixed greens.
4. Stir and eat right away.

65. **Delicious Chickpea Salad**

Servings 4

Preparation Time 15 minutes

INGREDIENTS

1. Chickpeas - 1 can, drained
2. Cherry tomatoes - 1 cup, quartered
3. Parsley - 1 2 cup, chopped
4. Red seedless grapes - 1 2 cup, halved
5. Feta cheese - 4 oz., cubed
6. Salt and pepper - to taste
7. Lemon juice - 1 tbsp.
8. Greek yogurt - 1 4 cup
9. Extra virgin olive oil - 2 tbsp.

DIRECTIONS

1. In a salad bowl, mix together parsley, chickpeas, grapes, feta cheese and tomatoes.
2. Add in remaining Ingredients:, seasoning with salt and pepper to suit your taste.
3. This fresh salad is best when served right away.

66. **Couscous Arugula Salad**

Servings 4

Preparation and Cooking Time 20 minutes

INGREDIENTS

- Couscous - 1 2 cup
- Vegetable stock - 1 cup
- Asparagus - 1 bunch, peeled
- Lemon - 1, juiced
- Dried tarragon - 1 tsp.
- Arugula - 2 cups
- Salt and pepper - to taste

DIRECTIONS

1. Heat vegetable stock in a pot until hot. Remove from heat and add in couscous. Cover until couscous has absorbed all the stock.
2. Pour in a bowl and fluff with a fork and then set aside to cool.
3. Peel asparagus with a vegetable peeler, making them into ribbons and put into a bowl with couscous.
4. Add remaining Ingredients and add salt and pepper to suit your taste.
5. Serve the salad immediately.

67. **Spinach and Grilled Feta Salad**

Servings 6

Preparation and Cooking Time 20 minutes

INGREDIENTS

- Feta cheese - 8 oz., sliced
- Black olives - 1 4 cup, sliced
- Green olives - 1 4 cup, sliced
- Baby spinach - 4 cups
- Garlic cloves - 2, minced
- Capers - 1 tsp., chopped
- Extra virgin olive oil - 2 tbsp.
- Red wine vinegar - 1 tbsp.

DIRECTIONS

1. Grill feta cheese slices over medium to high flame until brown on both sides.
2. In a salad bowl, mix green olives, black olives and spinach.
3. In a separate bowl, mix vinegar, capers and oil together to make a dressing.
4. Top salad with the dressing and cheese and it's is ready to serve.

68. **Creamy Cool Salad**

Servings 4

Preparation Time 15 minutes

INGREDIENTS

- Greek yogurt - 1 2 cup
- Dill - 2 tbsp., chopped
- Lemon juice - 1 tsp.
- Cucumbers - 4, diced
- Garlic cloves - 2, minced
- Salt and pepper - to taste

DIRECTIONS

1. Mix all Ingredients in a salad bowl.
2. Add salt and pepper to suit your taste and eat.

69. **Grilled Salmon Summer Salad**

Servings 4

Preparation and Cooking Time 30 minutes

INGREDIENTS

- Salmon fillets - 2

- Salt and pepper - to taste
- Vegetable stock - 2 cups
- Bulgur - 1 2 cup
- Cherry tomatoes - 1 cup, halved
- Sweet corn - 1 2 cup
- Lemon - 1, juiced
- Green olives - 1 2 cup, sliced
- Cucumber - 1, cubed
- Green onion - 1, chopped
- Red pepper - 1, chopped
- Red bell pepper - 1, cored and diced

DIRECTIONS

1. Heat a grill pan on medium and then place salmon on, seasoning with salt and pepper. Grill both sides of salmon until brown and set aside.
2. Heat stock in sauce pan until hot and then add in bulgur and cook until liquid is completely soaked into bulgur.
3. Mix salmon, bulgur and all other Ingredients in a salad bowl and again add salt and pepper, if desired, to suit your taste.
4. Serve salad as soon as completed.

70. **Broccoli Salad with Caramelized Onions**

Servings 4

Preparation and Cooking Time 25 minutes

INGREDIENTS

- Extra virgin olive oil - 3 tbsp.
- Red onions - 2, sliced
- Dried thyme - 1 tsp.
- Balsamic vinegar - 2 tbsp. vinegar
- Broccoli - 1 lb., cut into florets

- Salt and pepper - to taste

DIRECTIONS

1. Heat extra virgin olive oil in a pan over high heat and add in sliced onions. Cook for approximately 10 minutes or until the onions are caramelized. Stir in vinegar and thyme and then remove from stove.
2. Mix together the broccoli and onion mixture in a bowl, adding salt and pepper if desired. Serve and eat salad as soon as possible.

71. **Baked Cauliflower Mixed Salad**

Servings 4

Preparation and Cooking Time 30 minutes

INGREDIENTS

- Cauliflower - 1 lb., cut into florets
- Extra virgin olive oil - 2 tbsp.
- Dried mint - 1 tsp.
- Dried oregano - 1 tsp.
- Parsley - 2 tbsp., chopped
- Red pepper - 1, chopped
- Lemon - 1, juiced
- Green onion - 1, chopped
- Cilantro - 2 tbsp., chopped
- Salt and pepper to taste

DIRECTIONS

1. Heat oven to 350 degrees.
2. In a deep baking pan, combine olive oil, mint, cauliflower and oregano and bake for 15 minutes.
3. Once cooked, pour into a salad bowl and add remaining Ingredients:, stirring together.

4. Plate the salad and eat fresh and warm.

72. Quick Arugula Salad

Servings 4

Preparation Time 15 minutes

INGREDIENTS

- Roasted red bell peppers - 6, sliced
- Pine nuts - 2 tbsp.
- Dried raisins - 2 tbsp.
- Red onion - 1, sliced
- Arugula - 3 cups
- Balsamic vinegar - 2 tbsp.
- Feta cheese - 4 oz., crumbled
- Extra virgin olive oil – 2 tbsp.
- Feta cheese - 4 oz., crumbled
- Salt and pepper - to taste

DIRECTIONS

1. Using a salad bowl, combine vinegar, olive oil, pine nuts, raisins, peppers and onions.
2. Add arugula and feta cheese to the mix and serve.

73. Bell Pepper and Tomato Salad

Servings 4

Preparation Time 15 minutes

INGREDIENTS

- Roasted red bell pepper - 8, sliced
- Extra virgin olive oil - 2 tbsp.
- Chili flakes - 1 pinch
- Garlic cloves - 4, minced
- Pine nuts - 2 tbsp.

- Shallot - 1, sliced
- Cherry tomatoes - 1 cup, halved
- Parsley - 2 tbsp., chopped
- Balsamic vinegar - 1 tbsp.
- Salt and pepper - to taste

DIRECTIONS

1. Mix all Ingredients except salt and pepper in a salad bowl.
2. Season with salt and pepper if you want, to suit your taste.
3. Eat once freshly made.

74. One Bowl Spinach Salad

Servings 4

Preparation Time 20 minutes

INGREDIENTS

- Red beets - 2, cooked and diced
- Apple cider vinegar - 1 tbsp.
- Baby spinach - 3 cups
- Greek yogurt - 1 4 cup
- Horseradish - 1 tbsp.
- Salt and pepper - to taste

DIRECTIONS

1. Mix beets and spinach in a salad bowl.
2. Add in yogurt, horseradish, and vinegar. You can also add salt and pepper if you wish.
3. Serve salad as soon as mixed.

75. Olive and Red Bean Salad

Servings 4

Preparation Time 20 minutes

45

INGREDIENTS

- Red onions - 2, sliced
- Garlic cloves - 2, minced
- Balsamic vinegar - 2 tbsp.
- Green olives - 1 4 cup, sliced
- Salt and pepper - to taste
- Mixed greens - 2 cups
- Red beans - 1 can, drained
- Chili flakes - 1 pinch
- Extra virgin olive oil - 2 tbsp.
- Parsley - 2 tbsp., chopped

DIRECTIONS

- In a salad bowl, mix all Ingredients
- Add salt and pepper, if desired, and serve right away.

76. **Fresh and Light Cabbage Salad**

Servings 4

Preparation Time 25 minutes

INGREDIENTS

- Mint - 1 tbsp., chopped
- Ground coriander - 1 2 tsp.
- Savoy cabbage - 1, shredded
- Greek yogurt - 1 2 cup
- Cumin seeds - 1 4 tsp.
- Extra virgin olive oil - 2 tbsp.
- Carrot - 1, grated
- Red onion – 1, sliced
- Honey - 1 tsp.
- Lemon zest - 1 tsp.
- Lemon juice - 2 tbsp.
- Salt and pepper - to taste

DIRECTIONS

1. In a salad bowl, mix all Ingredients
2. You can add salt and pepper to suit your taste and then mix again.
3. This salad is best when cool and freshly made.

77. **Vegetable Patch Salad**

Servings 6

Preparation and Cooking Time 30 minutes

INGREDIENTS

- Cauliflower - 1 bunch, cut into florets
- Zucchini - 1, sliced
- Sweet potato - 1, peeled and cubed
- Baby carrots - 1 2 lb.
- Salt and pepper - to taste
- Dried basil - 1 tsp.
- Red onions - 2, sliced
- Eggplant - 2, cubed
- Endive - 1, sliced
- Extra virgin olive oil - 3 tbsp.
- Lemon – 1, juiced
- Balsamic vinegar - 1 tbsp.

DIRECTIONS

1. Preheat oven to 350 degrees. Mix together all vegetables, basil, salt, pepper and oil in a baking dish and cook for 25 – 30 minutes.
2. After cooked, pour into salad bowl and stir in vinegar and lemon juice.
3. Dish up and serve.

78. Cucumber Greek yoghurt Salad

Serves:6/

Preparation time: 5 minutes/

Cooking Time: 0 minutes

INGREDIENTS

- 4tbsp Greek yoghurt
- 4 large cucumbers peeled seeded and sliced
- 1 tbsp dried dill
- 1 tbsp apple cider vinegar
- 1/4 tsp garlic powder
- 1/4 tsp ground black pepper
- 1/2 tsp sugar
- 1/2 tsp salt

DIRECTIONS

1. Place all the Ingredients leaving out the cucumber into a bowl and whisk this until all is incorporated. Add your cucumber slices and toss until all is well mixed.
2. Let the salad chill 10 minutes in the refrigerator and then serve.

79. Chickpea Salad Recipe

Servings: 4 Duration: 15 minutes

INGREDIENTS

- Drained chickpeas: 1 can
- Halved cherry tomatoes: 1 cup
- Sun-dried chopped tomatoes: 1 2 cups
- Arugula: 2 cups
- Cubed pita bread: 1
- Pitted black olives: 1 2 cups

- 1 sliced shallot
- Cumin seeds: 1 2 teaspoon
- Coriander seeds: 1 2 teaspoon
- Chili powder: 1 4 teaspoon
- Chopped mint: 1 teaspoon
- Pepper and salt to taste
- Crumbled goat cheese: 4 oz.

DIRECTIONS

1. In a salad bowl, mix the tomatoes, chickpeas, pita bread, arugula, olives, shallot, spices and mint.
2. Stir in pepper and salt as desired to the cheese and stir.
3. You can now serve the fresh Salad.

80. Orange salad

Servings: 4

Cooking Time: 15 minutes

INGREDIENTS

- 4 sliced endives
- 1 sliced red onion
- 2 oranges already cut into segments
- Extra virgin olive oil: 2 tablespoon
- Pepper and salt to taste

DIRECTIONS

1. Mix all the Ingredients in a salad bowl
2. Sprinkle pepper and salt to taste.
3. You can now serve the salad fresh.

81. Yogurt lettuce salad recipe

Servings: 4

Cooking Time: 20 minutes

INGREDIENTS

- Shredded Romaine lettuce: 1 head
- Sliced cucumbers: 2
- 2 minced garlic cloves
- Greek yogurt: 1 2 cup
- Dijon mustard: 1 teaspoon
- Chili powder: 1 pinch
- Extra virgin olive oil: 2 tablespoon
- Lemon juice: 1 tablespoon
- Chopped dill: 2 tablespoon
- 4 chopped mint leaves
- Pepper and salt to taste

DIRECTIONS

1. In a salad bowl, combine the lettuce with the cucumbers.
2. Add the yogurt, chili, mustard, lemon juice, dill, mint, garlic and oil in a mortar with pepper and salt as desired. Then, mix well into paste, this is the dressing for the salad .
3. Top the Salad with the dressing then serve fresh.

82. **Fruit de salad recipe**

Servings: 4

Cooking Time: 20 minutes

INGREDIENTS

- Cubed seedless watermelon: 8 oz.
- Halved red grapes: 4 oz.
- 2 Sliced cucumbers
- Halved strawberries: 1 cup
- Cubed feta cheese: 6 oz.
- Balsamic vinegar: 2 tablespoon
- Arugula: 2 cups

DIRECTIONS

1. In a salad bowl, mix the strawberries, grapes, arugula, cucumbers, feta cheese and watermelon together.
2. Top the salad with vinegar and serve fresh.

83. **Chickpea with mint salad recipe**

Servings: 6 Duration: 20 minutes

INGREDIENTS

- 1 diced cucumber
- Sliced black olives:1 4 cup
- Chopped mint: 2 tablespoon
- Cooked and drained short pasta: 4 oz.
- Arugula: 2 cups
- Drained chickpeas: 1 can
- 1 sliced shallot
- Chopped Parsley: 1 2 cup
- Halved cherry tomatoes: 1 2 pound
- Sliced green olives: 1 4 cup
- 1 juiced lemon
- Extra virgin olive oil: 2 tablespoon
- Chopped walnut: 1 2 cup
- Pepper and salt to taste

DIRECTIONS

1. Mix the chickpeas with the other Ingredients in a salad bowl
2. Top with oil and lemon juice, sprinkle pepper and salt then mix well.
3. Refrigerate the Salad (can last in a sealed container for about 2 days) or serve fresh.

84. Grapy Fennel salad

Servings: 2 Time to prepare : 15 minutes

INGREDIENTS

- Grape seed oil: 1 tablespoon
- Chopped dill: 1 tablespoon
- 1 finely sliced fennel bulb
- Toasted almond slices: 2 tablespoon
- Chopped mint: 1 teaspoon
- 1 grapefruit already cut into segments
- 1 orange already cut into segments
- Pepper and salt as desired

DIRECTIONS

1. Using a platter, mix the grapefruit and orange segments with the fennel bulb
2. Add the mint, almond slices and dill, top with the oil and add pepper and salt as desired.
3. You can now serve the Salad fresh.

85. Greenie salad recipe

Servings: 4Duration: 15 minutes

INGREDIENTS

- Extra virgin olive oil: 2 tablespoon
- Mixed greens: 12 oz.
- Pitted black olives: 1 2 cup
- Pitted green olives: 1 4 cup
- Sherry vinegar: 2 tablespoon
- Pitted Kalamata olives: 1 2 cup
- Almond slices: 2 tablespoon
- Parmesan shavings: 2 oz.
- Sliced Parma ham: 2 oz.
- Pepper and salt as desired

DIRECTIONS

1. Stir the almonds, olives and mixed greens together in a salad bowl
2. Drizzle the oil and vinegar then sprinkle pepper and salt as you want.
3. Top with the Parma ham and Parmesan shavings before serving.
4. You can now serve fresh.

86. A Refreshing Detox Salad

Servings: 4,

Cooking Time: 0 minutes

INGREDIENTS

- 1 large apple, diced
- 1 large beet, coarsely grated
- 1 large carrot, coarsely grated
- 1 tbsp chia seeds
- 2 tbsp almonds, chopped
- 2 tbsp lemon juice
- 2 tbsp pumpkin seed oil
- 4 cups mixed greens

DIRECTIONS

1. In a medium salad bowl, except for mixed greens, combine all ingredients thoroughly.
2. Into 4 salad plates, divide the mixed greens.
3. Evenly top mixed greens with the salad bowl mixture.
4. Serve and enjoy.

NUTRITION:

Calories: 136.4; Protein: 1.93g; Carbs: 14.4g; Fat: 7.9g

87. Amazingly Fresh Carrot Salad

Servings: 4

Cooking Time: 0 minutes

INGREDIENTS

- ¼ tsp chipotle powder
- 1 bunch scallions, sliced
- 1 cup cherry tomatoes, halved
- 1 large avocado, diced
- 1 tbsp chili powder
- 1 tbsp lemon juice
- 2 tbsp olive oil
- 3 tbsp lime juice
- 4 cups carrots, spiralized
- salt to taste

DIRECTIONS

1. In a salad bowl, mix and arrange avocado, cherry tomatoes, scallions and spiralized carrots. Set aside.
2. In a small bowl, whisk salt, chipotle powder, chili powder, olive oil, lemon juice and lime juice thoroughly.
3. Pour dressing over noodle salad. Toss to coat well.
4. Serve and enjoy at room temperature.

NUTRITION:

Calories: 243.6; Fat: 14.8g; Protein: 3g; Carbs: 24.6g

88. Anchovy and Orange Salad

Servings: 4,

Cooking Time: 0 minutes

INGREDIENTS

- 1 small red onion, sliced into thin rounds
- 1 tbsp fresh lemon juice
- 1/8 tsp pepper or more to taste
- 16 oil cure Kalamata olives
- 2 tsp finely minced fennel fronds for garnish
- 3 tbsp extra virgin olive oil
- 4 small oranges, preferably blood oranges
- 6 anchovy fillets

DIRECTIONS

1. With a paring knife, peel oranges including the membrane that surrounds it.
2. In a plate, slice oranges into thin circles and allow plate to catch the orange juices.
3. On serving plate, arrange orange slices on a layer.
4. Sprinkle oranges with onion, followed by olives and then anchovy fillets.
5. Drizzle with oil, lemon juice and orange juice.
6. Sprinkle with pepper.
7. Allow salad to stand for 30 minutes at room temperature to allow the flavors to develop.
8. To serve, garnish with fennel fronds and enjoy.

NUTRITION:

Calories: 133.9; Protein: 3.2 g; Carbs: 14.3g; Fat: 7.1g

89. Arugula with Blueberries 'n Almonds

Servings: 2,

Cooking Time: 0 minutes

INGREDIENTS

- ½ cup slivered almonds
- ½ cup blueberries, fresh
- 1 ripe red pear, sliced
- 1 shallot, minced
- 1 tsp minced garlic
- 1 tsp whole grain mustard
- 2 tbsp fresh lemon juice
- 3 tbsp extra virgin olive oil
- 6 cups arugula

DIRECTIONS

1. In a big mixing bowl, mix garlic, olive oil, lemon juice and mustard.
2. Once thoroughly mixed, add remaining ingredients.
3. Toss to coat.
4. Equally divide into two bowls, serve and enjoy.

NUTRITION:

Calories: 530.4; **Protein:** 6.1g; **Carbs:** 39.2g; **Fat:** 38.8g

90. Asian Peanut Sauce Over Noodle Salad

Servings: 4,

Cooking Time: 0 minutes

INGREDIENTS

- 1 cup shredded green cabbage
- 1 cup shredded red cabbage
- 1/4 cup chopped cilantro
- 1/4 cup chopped peanuts
- 1/4 cup chopped scallions
- 4 cups shiritake noodles (drained and rinsed)
- Asian Peanut Sauce Ingredients
- ¼ cup sugar free peanut butter
- ¼ teaspoon cayenne pepper
- ½ cup filtered water
- ½ teaspoon kosher salt
- 1 tablespoon fish sauce (or coconut aminos for vegan)
- 1 tablespoon granulated erythritol sweetener
- 1 tablespoon lime juice
- 1 tablespoon toasted sesame oil
- 1 tablespoon wheat-free soy sauce
- 1 teaspoon minced garlic
- 2 tablespoons minced ginger

DIRECTIONS

1. In a large salad bowl, combine all noodle salad ingredients and toss well to mix.
2. In a blender, mix all sauce ingredients and pulse until smooth and creamy.
3. Pour sauce over the salad and toss well to coat.
4. Evenly divide into four equal servings and enjoy.

Calories: 104; **Protein:** 7.0g; **Carbs:** 12.0g; **Fat:** 16.0g

91. Asian Salad with pistachios

Servings: 6

Cooking Time: 0

INGREDIENTS

- ¼ cup chopped pistachios
- ¼ cup green onions, sliced
- 1 bunch watercress, trimmed
- 1 cup red bell pepper, diced
- 2 cups medium sized fennel bulb, thinly sliced
- 2 tbsp vegetable oil
- 3 cups Asian pears, cut into matchstick size
- 3 tbsp fresh lime juice

DIRECTIONS

1. In a large salad bowl, mix pistachios, green onions, bell pepper, fennel, watercress and pears.
2. In a small bowl, mix vegetable oil and lime juice. Season with pepper and salt to taste.
3. Pour dressing to salad and gently mix before serving.

NUTRITION:

Calories: 160; Protein: 3g; Fat: 1g; Carbs: 16g

92. Balela Salad from the Middle East

Servings: 6,

Cooking Time: 0 minutes

INGREDIENTS

- 1 jalapeno, finely chopped (optional)
- 1/2 green bell pepper, cored and chopped
- 2 1/2 cups grape tomatoes, slice in halves
- 1/2 cup sun-dried tomatoes
- 1/2 cup freshly chopped parsley leaves
- 1/2 cup freshly chopped mint or basil leaves
- 1/3 cup pitted Kalamata olives
- 1/4 cup pitted green olives
- 3 1/2 cups cooked chickpeas, drained and rinsed
- 3–5 green onions, both white and green parts, chopped
- Dressing Ingredients
- 1 garlic clove, minced
- 1 tsp ground sumac
- 1/2 tsp Aleppo pepper
- 1/4 cup Early Harvest Greek extra virgin olive oil
- 1/4 to 1/2 tsp crushed red pepper (optional)
- 2 tbsp lemon juice
- 2 tbsp white wine vinegar
- Salt and black pepper, a generous pinch to your taste

DIRECTIONS

1. mix together the salad ingredients in a large salad bowl.
2. In a separate smaller bowl or jar, mix together the dressing ingredients.
3. Drizzle the dressing over the salad and gently toss to coat.
4. Set aside for 30 minutes to allow the flavors to mix.
5. Serve and enjoy.

Calories: 257; Carbs: 30.5g; Protein: 8.4g; Fats: 12.6g

93. Blue Cheese and Portobello Salad

Servings: 2,

Cooking Time: 15 minutes

INGREDIENTS

- ½ cup croutons
- 1 tbsp merlot wine
- 1 tbsp water
- 1 tsp minced garlic
- 1 tsp olive oil
- 2 large Portobello mushrooms, stemmed, wiped clean and cut into bite sized pieces
- 2 pieces roasted red peppers (canned), sliced
- 2 tbsp balsamic vinegar
- 2 tbsp crumbled blue cheese
- 4 slices red onion
- 6 asparagus stalks cut into 1-inch sections
- 6 cups Bibb lettuce, chopped
- Ground pepper to taste

DIRECTIONS

1. On medium fire, place a small pan and heat oil. Once hot, add onions and mushrooms. For 4 to 6 minutes, sauté until tender.
2. Add garlic and for a minute continue sautéing.
3. Pour in wine and cook for a minute.
4. Bring an inch of water to a boil in a pot with steamer basket. Once boiling, add asparagus, steam for two to three minutes or until crisp and tender, while covered. Once cooked, remove basket from pot and set aside.
5. In a small bowl whisk thoroughly black pepper, water, balsamic vinegar, and blue cheese.
6. To serve, place 3 cups of lettuce on each plate. Add 1 roasted pepper, ½ of asparagus, ½ of mushroom mixture,

whisk blue cheese dressing before drizzling equally on to plates. Garnish with croutons, serve and enjoy.

NUTRITION: Calories: 660.8; **Protein:** 38.5g; **Carbs:** 30.4g; **Fat:** 42.8g

94. Blue Cheese and Arugula Salad

Servings: 4,

Cooking Time: 0 minutes

INGREDIENTS

- ¼ cup crumbled blue cheese
- 1 tsp Dijon mustard
- 1-pint fresh figs, quartered
- 2 bags arugula
- 3 tbsp Balsamic Vinegar
- 3 tbsp olive oil
- Pepper and salt to taste

DIRECTIONS

1. Whisk thoroughly together pepper, salt, olive oil, Dijon mustard, and balsamic vinegar to make the dressing. Set aside in the ref for at least 30 minutes to marinate and allow the spices to combine.
2. On four serving plates, evenly arrange arugula and top with blue cheese and figs.
3. Drizzle each plate of salad with 1 ½ tbsp of prepared dressing.
4. Serve and enjoy.

NUTRITION: Calories: 202; **Protein:** 2.5g; **Carbs:** 25.5g; **Fat:** 10g

95. Broccoli Salad Moroccan Style

Servings: 4,

Cooking Time: 0 minutes

INGREDIENTS

- ¼ tsp sea salt
- ¼ tsp ground cinnamon
- ½ tsp ground turmeric
- ¾ tsp ground ginger
- ½ tbsp extra virgin olive oil
- ½ tbsp apple cider vinegar
- 2 tbsp chopped green onion
- 1/3 cup coconut cream
- ½ cup carrots, shredded
- 1 small head of broccoli, chopped

DIRECTIONS

1. In a large salad bowl, mix well salt, cinnamon, turmeric, ginger, olive oil, and vinegar.
2. Add remaining ingredients, tossing well to coat.
3. Pop in the ref for at least 30 to 60 minutes before serving.

NUTRITION: Calories: 90.5; Protein: 1.3g; Carbs: 4g; Fat: 7.7g

96. **Charred Tomato and Broccoli Salad**

Servings: 6,

Cooking Time: minutes

INGREDIENTS

- ¼ cup lemon juice
- ½ tsp chili powder
- 1 ½ lbs. boneless chicken breast
- 1 ½ lbs. medium tomato
- 1 tsp freshly ground pepper

- 1 tsp salt
- 4 cups broccoli florets
- 5 tbsp extra virgin olive oil, divided to 2 and 3 tablespoons

DIRECTIONS

1. Place the chicken in a skillet and add just enough water to cover the chicken. Bring to a simmer over high heat. Reduce the heat once the liquid boils and cook the chicken thoroughly for 12 minutes. Once cooked, shred the chicken into bite-sized pieces.
2. On a large pot, bring water to a boil and add the broccoli. Cook for 5 minutes until slightly tender. Drain and rinse the broccoli with cold water. Set aside.
3. Core the tomatoes and cut them crosswise. Discard the seeds and set the tomatoes cut side down on paper towels. Pat them dry.
4. In a heavy skillet, heat the pan over high heat until very hot. Brush the cut sides of the tomatoes with olive oil and place them on the pan. Cook the tomatoes until the sides are charred. Set aside.
5. In the same pan, heat the remaining 3 tablespoon olive oil over medium heat. Stir the salt, chili powder and pepper and stir for 45 seconds. Pour over the lemon juice and remove the pan from the heat.
6. Plate the broccoli, shredded chicken and chili powder mixture dressing.

NUTRITION: Calories: 210.8; Protein: 27.5g; Carbs: 6.3g; Fat: 8.4g

97. Chopped Chicken on Greek Salad

Servings: 4,

Cooking Time: 0 minutes

INGREDIENTS

- ¼ tsp pepper
- ¼ tsp salt
- ½ cup crumbled feta cheese
- ½ cup finely chopped red onion
- ½ cup sliced ripe black olives
- 1 medium cucumber, peeled, seeded and chopped
- 1 tbsp chopped fresh dill
- 1 tsp garlic powder
- 1/3 cup red wine vinegar
- 2 ½ cups chopped cooked chicken
- 2 medium tomatoes, chopped
- 2 tbsp extra virgin olive oil
- 6 cups chopped romaine lettuce

DIRECTIONS

1. In a large bowl, whisk well pepper, salt, garlic powder, dill, oil and vinegar.
2. Add feta, olives, onion, cucumber, tomatoes, chicken, and lettuce.
3. Toss well to combine.
4. Serve and enjoy.

NUTRITION: Calories: 461.9; Protein: 19.4g; Carbs: 10.8g; Fat: 37.9g

98. Classic Greek Salad

Servings: 4,

Cooking Time: 0 minutes

INGREDIENTS

- ¼ cup extra virgin olive oil, plus more for drizzling
- ¼ cup red wine vinegar
- 1 4-oz block Greek feta cheese packed in brine
- 1 cup Kalamata olives, halved and pitted
- 1 lemon, juiced and zested
- 1 small red onion, halved and thinly sliced
- 1 tsp dried oregano
- 1 tsp honey
- 14 small vine-ripened tomatoes, quartered
- 5 Persian cucumbers
- Fresh oregano leaves for topping, optional
- Pepper to taste
- Salt to taste

DIRECTIONS

1. In a bowl of ice water, soak red onions with 2 tbsp salt.
2. In a large bowl, whisk well ¼ tsp pepper, ½ tsp salt, dried oregano, honey, lemon zest, lemon juice, and vinegar. Slowly pour olive oil in a steady stream as you briskly whisk mixture. Continue whisking until emulsified.
3. Add olives and tomatoes, toss to coat with dressing.
4. Alternatingly peel cucumber leaving strips of skin on. Trim ends slice lengthwise and chop in ½-inch thick cubes. Add into bowl of tomatoes.
5. Drain onions and add into bowl of tomatoes. Toss well to coat and mix.
6. Drain feta and slice into four equal rectangles.
7. Divide Greek salad into serving plates, top each with oregano and feta.

8. To serve, season with pepper and drizzle with oil and enjoy.

NUTRITION: Calories: 365.5; Protein: 9.6g; Carbs: 26.2g; Fat: 24.7g

99. Cold Zucchini Noodle Bowl

Servings: 4,

Cooking Time: 20 minutes

INGREDIENTS

- ¼ cup basil leaves, roughly chopped
- ¼ cup olive oil
- ¼ tsp sea salt
- ½ tsp salt1 tsp garlic powder
- 1 lb. peeled and uncooked shrimp
- 1 tsp lemon zest
- 1 tsp lime zest
- 2 tbsp butter
- 2 tbsp lemon juice
- 2 tbsp lime juice
- 3 clementine, peeled and separated
- 4 cups zucchini, spirals or noodles
- pinch of black pepper

DIRECTIONS

1. Make zucchini noodles and set aside.
2. On medium fire, place a large nonstick saucepan and heat butter.
3. Meanwhile, pat dry shrimps and season with salt and garlic. Add into hot saucepan and sauté for 6 minutes or until opaque and cooked.
4. Remove from pan, transfer to a bowl and put aside.
5. Right away, add zucchini noodles to still hot pan and stir fry for a minute. Leave noodles on pan as you prepare the dressing.

6. Blend well salt, olive oil, juice and zest in a small bowl.
7. Then place noodles into salad bowl, top with shrimp, pour oil mixture, basil and clementine. Toss to mix well.
8. Refrigerate for an hour before serving.

NUTRITION: Calories: 353.4; Carbs: 14.8g; Protein: 24.5g; Fat: 21.8g

100. Coleslaw Asian Style

Servings: 10

Cooking Time: 0 minutes

INGREDIENTS

- ½ cup chopped fresh cilantro
- 1 ½ tbsp minced garlic
- 2 carrots, julienned
- 2 cups shredded napa cabbage
- 2 cups thinly sliced red cabbage
- 2 red bell peppers, thinly sliced
- 2 tbsp minced fresh ginger root
- 3 tbsp brown sugar
- 3 tbsp soy sauce
- 5 cups thinly sliced green cabbage
- 5 tbsp creamy peanut butter
- 6 green onions, chopped
- 6 tbsp rice wine vinegar
- 6 tbsp vegetable oil

DIRECTIONS

1. Mix thoroughly the following in a medium bowl: garlic, ginger, brown sugar, soy sauce, peanut butter, oil and rice vinegar.
2. In a separate bowl, blend well cilantro, green onions, carrots, bell pepper, Napa cabbage, red cabbage and green cabbage. Pour in the peanut sauce above and toss to mix well.

3. Serve and enjoy.

NUTRITION: Calories: 193.8; Protein: 4g; Fat: 12.6g; Carbs: 16.1g

101. Cucumber and Tomato Salad

Servings: 4,

Cooking Time: 0 minutes

INGREDIENTS

- Ground pepper to taste
- Salt to taste
- 1 tbsp fresh lemon juice
- 1 onion, chopped
- 1 cucumber, peeled and diced
- 2 tomatoes, chopped
- 4 cups spinach

DIRECTIONS

1. In a salad bowl, mix onions, cucumbers and tomatoes.
2. Season with pepper and salt to taste.
3. Add lemon juice and mix well.
4. Add spinach, toss to coat, serve and enjoy.

NUTRITION: Calories: 70.3; Fat: 0.3g; Protein: 1.3g; Carbohydrates: 7.1g

102. Cucumber Salad Japanese Style

Servings: 5 servings

Cooking Time: 0 minutes

INGREDIENTS

- 1 ½ tsp minced fresh ginger root
- 1 tsp salt
- 1/3 cup rice vinegar
- 2 large cucumbers, ribbon cut
- 4 tsp white sugar

DIRECTIONS

1. Mix well ginger, salt, sugar and vinegar in a small bowl.
2. Add ribbon cut cucumbers and mix well.
3. Let stand for at least one hour in the ref before serving.

NUTRITION: Calories: 29; Fat: .2g; Protein: .7g; Carbs: 6.1g

103. Easy Garden Salad with Arugula

Servings: 2

Cooking Time: 0

INGREDIENTS

- ¼ cup grated parmesan cheese
- ¼ cup pine nuts
- 1 cup cherry tomatoes, halved
- 1 large avocado, sliced into ½ inch cubes
- 1 tbsp rice vinegar
- 2 tbsp olive oil or grapeseed oil
- 4 cups young arugula leaves, rinsed and dried
- Black pepper, freshly ground
- Salt to taste

DIRECTIONS

1. Get a bowl with cover, big enough to hold the salad and mix together the parmesan cheese, vinegar, oil, pine nuts, cherry tomatoes and arugula.

2. Season with pepper and salt according to how you like it. Place the lid and jiggle the covered bowl to combine the salad.
3. Serve the salad topped with sliced avocadoes.

NUTRITION: Calories: 490.8; Fat: 43.6g; Protein: 9.1g; Carbs: 15.5g

104. Easy Quinoa & Pear Salad

Servings: 6,

Cooking Time: 0 minutes

INGREDIENTS

- ¼ cup chopped parsley
- ¼ cup chopped scallions
- ¼ cup lime juice
- ¼ cup red onion, diced
- ½ cup diced carrots
- ½ cup diced celery
- ½ cup diced cucumber
- ½ cup diced red pepper
- ½ cup dried wild blueberries
- ½ cup olive oil
- ½ cup spicy pecans, chopped
- 1 tbsp chopped parsley
- 1 tsp honey
- 1 tsp sea salt
- 2 fresh pears, cut into chunks
- 3 cups cooked quinoa

DIRECTIONS

1. In a small bowl mix well olive oil, salt, lime juice, honey, and parsley. Set aside.
2. In large salad bowl, add remaining ingredients and toss to mix well.
3. Pour dressing and toss well to coat.

4. Serve and enjoy.

NUTRITION: Calories: 382; Protein: 5.6g; Carbs: 31.4g; Fat: 26g

105. Easy-Peasy Club Salad

Servings: 3,

Cooking Time: 0 minutes

INGREDIENTS

- ½ cup cherry tomatoes, halved
- ½ teaspoon garlic powder
- ½ teaspoon onion powder
- 1 cup diced cucumber
- 1 tablespoon Dijon mustard
- 1 tablespoon milk
- 1 teaspoon dried parsley
- 2 tablespoons mayonnaise
- 2 tablespoons sour cream
- 3 cups romaine lettuce, torn into pieces
- 3 large hard-boiled eggs, sliced
- 4 ounces cheddar cheese, cubed

DIRECTIONS

1. Make the dressing by mixing garlic powder, onion powder, dried parsley, mayonnaise, and sour cream in a small bowl. Add a tablespoon of milk and mix well. If you want the dressing thinner, you can add more milk.
2. In a salad platter, layer salad ingredients with Dijon mustard in the middle.
3. Evenly drizzle with dressing and toss well to coat.
4. Serve and enjoy.

NUTRITION: Calories: 335.5; Protein: 16.8g; Carbs: 7.9g; Fat: 26.3g

106. <u>Fennel and Seared Scallops Salad</u>

Servings: 4,

Cooking Time: 10 minutes

INGREDIENTS

- ¼ tsp salt
- ½ large fennel bulb, halved, cored and very thinly sliced
- ½ tsp whole fennel seeds, freshly ground
- 1 large pink grapefruit
- 1 lb. fresh sea scallops, muscle removed, room temperature
- 1 tbsp olive oil, divided
- 1 tsp raw honey
- 12 whole almonds chopped coarsely and lightly toasted
- 4 cups red leaf lettuce, cored and torn into bite sized pieces
- A pinch of ground pepper

DIRECTIONS

1. To catch the juices, work over a bowl. Peel and segment grapefruit. Strain the juice in a cup.
2. For the dressing, whisk together in a small bowl black pepper, 1/8 tsp salt, 1/8 tsp ground fennel, honey, 2 tsp water, 2 tsp oil and 3 tbsp of pomegranate juice. Set aside 1 tbsp of the dressing.
3. Pat scallops dry with a paper towel and season with remaining salt and ½ tsp ground fennel.
4. On medium fire, place a nonstick skillet and brush with 1 tsp oil. Once heated, add ½ of scallops and cook until lightly browned or for 5 minutes

each side. Transfer to a plate and keep warm as you cook the second batch using the same process.

5. Mix together dressing, lettuce and fennel in a large salad bowl. Divide evenly onto 4 salad plates.
6. Evenly top each salad with scallops, grapefruit segments and almonds. Drizzle with reserved dressing, serve and enjoy.

NUTRITION: Calories: 231.9; **Protein:** 25.3g; Carbs: 18.5g; Fat: 6.3g

107. <u>Fruity Asparagus-Quinoa Salad</u>

Servings: 8,

Cooking Time: 25 minutes

INGREDIENTS

- ¼ cup chopped pecans, toasted
- ½ cup finely chopped white onion
- ½ jalapeno pepper, diced
- ½ lb. asparagus, sliced to 2-inch lengths, steamed and chilled
- ½ tsp kosher salt
- 1 cup fresh orange sections
- 1 cup uncooked quinoa
- 1 tsp olive oil
- 2 cups water
- 2 tbsp minced red onion
- 5 dates, pitted and chopped

Dressing ingredients

- ¼ tsp ground black pepper
- ¼ tsp kosher salt
- 1 garlic clove, minced
- 1 tbsp olive oil
- 2 tbsp chopped fresh mint

- 2 tbsp fresh lemon juice
- Mint sprigs – optional

DIRECTIONS

1. Wash and rub with your hands the quinoa in a bowl at least three times, discarding water each and every time.
2. On medium high fire, place a large nonstick fry pan and heat 1 tsp olive oil. For two minutes, sauté onions before adding quinoa and sautéing for another five minutes.
3. Add ½ tsp salt and 2 cups water and bring to a boil. Lower fire to a simmer, cover and cook for 15 minutes. Turn off fire and let stand until water is absorbed.
4. Add pepper, asparagus, dates, pecans and orange sections into a salad bowl. Add cooked quinoa, toss to mix well.
5. In a small bowl, whisk mint, garlic, black pepper, salt, olive oil and lemon juice to create the dressing.
6. Pour dressing over salad, serve and enjoy.

NUTRITION: Calories: 173; Fat: 6.3g; Protein: 4.3g; Carbohydrates: 24.7g

108. Garden Salad with Balsamic Vinegar

Servings: 1,

Cooking Time: 0 minutes

INGREDIENTS

- 1 cup baby arugula
- 1 cup spinach
- 1 tbsp craisins
- 1 tbsp almonds, shaved or chopped
- 1 tbsp balsamic vinegar
- ½ tbsp extra virgin olive oil

DIRECTIONS

1. In a plate, mix arugula and spinach.
2. Top with craisins and almonds.
3. Drizzle olive oil and balsamic vinegar.
4. Serve and enjoy.

NUTRITION: Calories: 206; Fat: 15 g; Protein: 5g; Carbohydrates: 14g

109. Garden Salad with Oranges and Olives

Servings: 4

Cooking Time: 15 minutes

INGREDIENTS

- ½ cup red wine vinegar
- 1 tbsp extra virgin olive oil
- 1 tbsp finely chopped celery
- 1 tbsp finely chopped red onion
- 16 large ripe black olives
- 2 garlic cloves
- 2 navel oranges, peeled and segmented
- 4 boneless, skinless chicken breasts, 4-oz each
- 4 garlic cloves, minced
- 8 cups leaf lettuce, washed and dried
- Cracked black pepper to taste

DIRECTIONS

- Prepare the dressing by mixing pepper, celery, onion, olive oil, garlic and vinegar in a small bowl. Whisk well to combine.
- Lightly grease grate and preheat grill to high.

- Rub chicken with the garlic cloves and discard garlic.
- Grill chicken for 5 minutes per side or until cooked through.
- Remove from grill and let it stand for 5 minutes before cutting into ½-inch strips.
- In 4 serving plates, evenly arrange two cups lettuce, ¼ of the sliced oranges and 4 olives per plate.
- Top each plate with ¼ serving of grilled chicken, evenly drizzle with dressing, serve and enjoy.

NUTRITION: Calories: 259.8; Protein: 48.9g; Carbs: 12.9g; Fat: 1.4g

110. <u>**Garden Salad with Grapes**</u>

Servings: 6,

Cooking Time: 0 minutes

INGREDIENTS

- ¼ tsp black pepper
- ¼ tsp salt
- ½ tsp stone-ground mustard
- 1 tsp chopped fresh thyme
- 1 tsp honey
- 1 tsp maple syrup
- 2 cups red grapes, halved
- 2 tbsp toasted sunflower seed kernels
- 2 tsp grapeseed oil
- 3 tbsp red wine vinegar
- 7 cups loosely packed baby arugula

DIRECTIONS

1. In a small bowl whisk together mustard, syrup, honey and vinegar. Whisking continuously, slowly add oil.

2. In a large salad bowl, mix thyme, seeds, grapes and arugula.
3. Drizzle with the oil dressing, season with pepper and salt.
4. Gently toss to coat salad with the dressing.

NUTRITION: Calories: 85.7; Protein: 1.6g; Carbs: 12.4g; Fat: 3.3g

111. <u>**Ginger Yogurt Dressed Citrus Salad**</u>

Servings: 6,

Cooking Time: minutes

INGREDIENTS

- 2/3 cup minced crystallized ginger
- 1 16-oz Greek yogurt
- ¼ tsp ground cinnamon
- 2 tbsp honey
- ½ cup dried cranberries
- 3 navel oranges
- 2 large tangerines, peeled
- 1 pink grapefruit, peeled

DIRECTIONS

1. Into sections, break tangerines and grapefruit.
2. Cut tangerine sections into half.
3. Into thirds, slice grapefruit sections.
4. Cut orange pith and peel in half and slice oranges into ¼ inch thick rounds, then quartered.
5. In a medium bowl, mix oranges, grapefruit, tangerines and its juices.
6. Add cinnamon, honey and ½ cup of cranberries.
7. Cover and place in the ref for an hour.
8. In a small bowl, mix ginger and yogurt.

9. To serve, add a dollop of yogurt dressing onto a serving of fruit and sprinkle with cranberries.

NUTRITION: Calories: 190; Protein: 2.9g; Carbs: 16.7g; Fat: 12.4g

112. Goat Cheese and Oregano Dressing Salad

Servings: 4,

Cooking Time: 0 minutes

INGREDIENTS

- ¾ cup crumbled soft fresh goat cheese
- 1 ½ cups diced celery
- 1 ½ large red bell peppers, diced
- 1 tbsp chopped fresh oregano
- 1/3 cup chopped red onion
- 2 tbsp extra virgin olive oil
- 2 tbsp fresh lemon juice
- 4 cups baby spinach leaves, coarsely chopped

DIRECTIONS

1. In a large salad bowl, mix oregano, lemon juice and oil.
2. Add pepper and salt to taste.
3. Mix in red onion, goat cheese, celery, bell peppers and spinach.
4. Toss to coat well, serve and enjoy. Ingredients

NUTRITION: Calories: 110.9; Protein: 6.9g; Carbs: 10.7g; Fat: 4.5g

113. Grape and Walnut Garden Salad

Servings: 2,

Cooking Time: 0 minutes

INGREDIENTS

- ½ cup chopped walnuts, toasted
- 1 ripe persimmon
- ½ cup red grapes, halved lengthwise
- 1 shallot, minced
- 1 tsp minced garlic
- 1 tsp whole grain mustard
- 2 tbsp fresh lemon juice
- 3 tbsp extra virgin olive oil
- 6 cups baby spinach

DIRECTIONS

1. Cut persimmon and red pear into ½-inch cubes. Discard seeds.
2. In a medium bowl, whisk garlic, shallot, olive oil, lemon juice and mustard to make the dressing.
3. In a medium salad bowl, toss to mix spinach, pear and persimmon.
4. Pour in dressing and toss to coat well.
5. Garnish with pecans.
6. Serve and enjoy.

NUTRITION: Calories: 440; Protein: 6.1g; Carbs: 39.1g; Fat: 28.8g

114. Greek Antipasto Salad

Servings: 4,

Cooking Time: 0 minutes

INGREDIENTS

- ½ cup artichoke hearts, chipped
- ½ cup olives, sliced
- ½ cup sweet peppers, roasted
- 1 large head romaine lettuce, chopped
- 4 ounces cooked prosciutto, cut into thin strips

- 4 ounces cooked salami, cubed
- Italian dressing to taste

DIRECTIONS

1. In a large mixing bowl, add all the ingredients except the Italian dressing. Mix everything until the vegetables are evenly distributed.
2. Add the Italian dressing and toss to combine.
3. Serve chilled.

NUTRITION: Calories: 425.8; Fat: 38.9 g; Protein: 39.2 g; Carbs: 12.6 g

115. **Grilled Halloumi Cheese Salad**

Servings: 1,

Cooking Time: 10 minutes

INGREDIENTS

- 0.5 oz chopped walnuts
- 1 handful baby arugula
- 1 Persian cucumber, sliced into circles about ½-inch thick
- 3 oz halloumi cheese
- 5 grape tomatoes, sliced in half
- balsamic vinegar
- olive oil
- salt

DIRECTIONS

1. Into 1/3 slices, cut the cheese. For 3 to 5 minutes each side, grill the kinds of cheese until you can see grill marks.
2. In a salad bowl, add arugula, cucumber, and tomatoes. Drizzle with olive oil and balsamic vinegar. Season with salt and toss well coat.
3. Sprinkle walnuts and add grilled halloumi.
4. Serve and enjoy.

NUTRITION: Calories: 543; Protein: 21.0g; Carbs: 9.0g; Fat: 47.0g

116. **Grilled Eggplant Salad**

Servings: 4,

Cooking Time: 18 minutes

INGREDIENTS

- 1 avocado, halved, pitted, peeled and cubed
- 1 Italian eggplant, cut into 1-inch thick slices
- 1 large red onion, cut into rounds
- 1 lemon, zested
- 1 tbsp coarsely chopped oregano leaves
- 1 tbsp red wine vinegar
- 1 tsp Dijon mustard
- Canola oil
- Freshly ground black pepper
- Honey
- Olive oil
- Parsley sprigs for garnish
- Salt

DIRECTIONS

1. With canola oil, brush onions and eggplant and place on grill.
2. Grill on high until onions are slightly charred and eggplants are soft around 5 minutes for onions and 8 to 12 minutes for eggplant.
3. Remove from grill and let cool for 5 minutes.

4. Roughly chop eggplants and onions and place in salad bowl.
5. Add avocado and toss to mix.
6. Whisk oregano, mustard and red wine vinegar in a small bowl.
7. Whisk in olive oil and honey to taste. Season with pepper and salt to taste.
8. Pour dressing to eggplant mixture, toss to mix well.
9. Garnish with parsley sprigs and lemon zest before serving.

NUTRITION: Calories: 190; Protein: 2.9g; Carbs: 16.7g; Fat: 12.4g

117. Grilled Vegetable Salad

Servings: 3

Cooking Time: 7 minutes

INGREDIENTS

- ¼ cup extra virgin olive oil, for brushing
- ¼ cup fresh basil leaves
- ¼ lb. feta cheese
- ½ bunch asparagus, trimmed and cut into bite-size pieces
- 1 medium onion, cut into ½ inch rings
- 1-pint cherry tomatoes
- 1 red bell pepper, quartered, seeds and ribs removed
- 1 yellow bell pepper, quartered, seeds and ribs removed
- Pepper and salt to taste

DIRECTIONS

- Toss olive oil and vegetables in a big bowl. Season with salt and pepper.
- Frill vegetables in a preheated griller for 5-7 minutes or until charred and tender.

- Transfer veggies to a platter, add feta and basil.
- In a separate small bowl, mix olive oil, balsamic vinegar, garlic seasoned with pepper and salt.
- Drizzle dressing over vegetables and serve.

NUTRITION: Calories: 147.6; Protein: 3.8g; Fat: 19.2g; Carbs: 13.9 g

118. Healthy Detox Salad

Servings: 4,

Cooking Time: 0 minutes

INGREDIENTS

- 4 cups mixed greens
- 2 tbsp lemon juice
- 2 tbsp pumpkin seed oil
- 1 tbsp chia seeds
- 2 tbsp almonds, chopped
- 1 large apple, diced
- 1 large carrot, coarsely grated
- 1 large beet, coarsely grated

DIRECTIONS

1. In a medium salad bowl, except for mixed greens, combine all ingredients thoroughly.
2. Into 4 salad plates, divide the mixed greens.
3. Evenly top mixed greens with the salad bowl mixture.
4. Serve and enjoy.

NUTRITION: Calories: 141; Protein: 2.1g; Carbs: 14.7g; Fat: 8.2g

119. Herbed Calamari Salad

Servings: 6,

Cooking Time: 25 minutes

INGREDIENTS

- ¼ cup finely chopped cilantro leaves
- ¼ cup finely chopped mint leaves
- ¼ tsp freshly ground black pepper
- ½ cup finely chopped flat leaf parsley leaves
- ¾ tsp kosher salt
- 2 ½ lbs. cleaned and trimmed uncooked calamari rings and tentacles, defrosted
- 3 medium garlic cloves, smashed and minced
- 3 tbsp extra virgin olive oil
- A pinch of crushed red pepper flakes
- Juice of 1 large lemon
- Peel of 1 lemon, thinly sliced into strips

DIRECTIONS

1. On a nonstick large fry pan, heat 1 ½ tbsp olive oil. Once hot, sauté garlic until fragrant around a minute.
2. Add calamari, making sure that they are in one layer, if pan is too small then cook in batches.
3. Season with pepper and salt, after 2 to 4 minutes of searing, remove calamari from pan with a slotted spoon and transfer to a large bowl. Continue cooking remainder of calamari.
4. Season cooked calamari with herbs, lemon rind, lemon juice, red pepper flakes, pepper, salt, and remaining olive oil.
5. Toss well to coat, serve and enjoy.

NUTRITION: Calories: 551.7; Protein: 7.3g; Carbs: 121.4g; Fat: 4.1g

120. <u>Herbed Chicken Salad Greek Style</u>

Servings: 6

Cooking Time: 0 minutes

INGREDIENTS

- ¼ cup or 1 oz crumbled feta cheese
- ½ tsp garlic powder
- ½ tsp salt
- ¾ tsp black pepper, divided
- 1 cup grape tomatoes, halved
- 1 cup peeled and chopped English cucumbers
- 1 cup plain fat-free yogurt
- 1 pound skinless, boneless chicken breast, cut into 1-inch cubes
- 1 tsp bottled minced garlic
- 1 tsp ground oregano
- 2 tsp sesame seed paste or tahini
- 5 tsp fresh lemon juice, divided
- 6 pitted kalamata olives, halved
- 8 cups chopped romaine lettuce
- Cooking spray

DIRECTIONS

1. In a bowl, mix together ¼ tsp salt, ½ tsp pepper, garlic powder and oregano. Then on medium high heat place a skillet and coat with cooking spray and sauté together the spice mixture and chicken until chicken is cooked. Before transferring to bowl, drizzle with juice.
2. In a small bowl, mix thoroughly the following: garlic, tahini, yogurt, ¼ tsp pepper, ¼ tsp salt, and 2 tsp juice.
3. In another bowl, mix together olives, tomatoes, cucumber and lettuce.

4. To Serve salad, place 2 ½ cups of lettuce mixture on plate, topped with ½ cup chicken mixture, 3 tbsp yogurt mixture and 1 tbsp of cheese.

NUTRITION: Calories: 170.1; Fat: 3.7g; Protein: 20.7g; Carbs: 13.5g

121. Kale Salad Recipe

Servings: 4,

Cooking Time: 7 minutes

INGREDIENTS

- ¼ cup Kalamata olives
- ½ of a lemon
- 1 ½ tbsp flaxseeds
- 1 garlic clove, minced
- 1 small cucumber, sliced thinly
- 1 tbsp extra virgin olive oil
- 2 tbsp green onion, chopped
- 2 tbsp red onion, minced
- 6 cups dinosaur kale, chopped
- a pinch of dried basil
- a pinch of salt

DIRECTIONS

1. Bring a medium pot, half-filled with water to a boil.
2. Rinse kale and cut into small strips. Place in a steamer and put on top of boiling water and steam for 5 – 7 minutes.
3. Transfer steamed kale to a salad bowl.
4. Season kale with oil, salt, basil and lemon. Toss to coat well.
5. Add remaining ingredients into salad bowl, toss to mix.
6. Serve and enjoy.

NUTRITION: Calories: 92.7; Protein: 2.4g; Carbs: 6.6g; Fat: 6.3g

122. Cheesy Keto Zucchini Soup

Servings: 2

Preparation time: 20 mins

INGREDIENTS

- ½ medium onion, peeled and chopped
- 1 cup bone broth
- 1 tablespoon coconut oil
- 1½ zucchinis, cut into chunks
- ½ tablespoon nutrition al yeast
- Dash of black pepper
- ½ tablespoon parsley, chopped, for garnish
- ½ tablespoon coconut cream, for garnish

DIRECTIONS

1. Melt the coconut oil in a large pan over medium heat and add onions.
2. Sauté for about 3 minutes and add zucchinis and bone broth.
3. Reduce the heat to simmer for about 15 minutes and cover the pan.
4. Add nutrition al yeast and transfer to an immersion blender.
5. Blend until smooth and season with black pepper.
6. Top with coconut cream and parsley to serve.

NUTRITION: Calories: 154 Carbs: 8.9g Fats: 8.1g Proteins: 13.4g Sodium: 93mg Sugar: 3.9g

123. Spring Soup with Poached Egg

Servings: 2

Preparation time: 20 mins

INGREDIENTS

- 32 oz vegetable broth
- 2 eggs
- 1 head romaine lettuce, chopped
- Salt, to taste

DIRECTIONS

1. Bring the vegetable broth to a boil and reduce the heat.
2. Poach the eggs for 5 minutes in the broth and remove them into 2 bowls.
3. Stir in romaine lettuce into the broth and cook for 4 minutes.
4. Dish out in a bowl and serve hot.

NUTRITION: Calories: 158 Carbs: 6.9g Fats: 7.3g Proteins: 15.4g Sodium: 1513mg Sugar: 3.3g

124. Mint Avocado Chilled Soup

Servings: 2

Preparation time: 15 mins

INGREDIENTS

- 2 romaine lettuce leaves
- 1 Tablespoon lime juice
- 1 medium ripe avocado
- 1 cup coconut milk, chilled
- 20 fresh mint leaves
- Salt to taste

DIRECTIONS

1. Put all the ingredients in a blender and blend until smooth.
2. Refrigerate for about 10 minutes and serve chilled.

NUTRITION: Calories: 432 Carbs: 16.1g Fats: 42.2g Proteins: 5.2g Sodium: 33mg Sugar: 4.5g

125. Easy Butternut Squash Soup

Servings: 4

Preparation time: 1 hour 45 mins

INGREDIENTS

- 1 small onion, chopped
- 4 cups chicken broth
- 1 butternut squash
- 3 tablespoons coconut oil
- Salt, to taste
- Nutmeg and pepper, to taste

DIRECTIONS

1. Put oil and onions in a large pot and add onions.
2. Sauté for about 3 minutes and add chicken broth and butternut squash.
3. Simmer for about 1 hour on medium heat and transfer into an immersion blender.
4. Pulse until smooth and season with salt, pepper and nutmeg.
5. Return to the pot and cook for about 30 minutes.
6. Dish out and serve hot.

NUTRITION: Calories: 149 Carbs: 6.6g Fats: 11.6g Proteins: 5.4g Sodium: 765mg Sugar: 2.2g

126. **Spring Soup Recipe with Poached Egg**

Servings: 2

Preparation time: 20 mins

INGREDIENTS

- 2 eggs
- 2 tablespoons butter
- 4 cups chicken broth
- 1 head of romaine lettuce, chopped
- Salt, to taste

DIRECTIONS

1. Boil the chicken broth and lower heat.
2. Poach the eggs in the broth for about 5 minutes and remove the eggs.
3. Place each egg into a bowl and add chopped romaine lettuce into the broth.
4. Cook for about 10 minutes and ladle the broth with the lettuce into the bowls.

NUTRITION: Calories: 264 Carbs: 7g Fats: 18.9g Proteins: 16.1g Sodium: 1679mg Sugar: 3.4g

127. **Cauliflower, leek & bacon soup**

Servings: 4

Preparation time: 10 mins

INGREDIENTS

- 4 cups chicken broth
- ½ cauliflower head, chopped
- 1 leek, chopped
- Salt and black pepper, to taste
- 5 bacon strips

DIRECTIONS

1. Put the cauliflower, leek and chicken broth into the pot and cook for about 1 hour on medium heat.
2. Transfer into an immersion blender and pulse until smooth.
3. Return the soup into the pot and microwave the bacon strips for 1 minute.
4. Cut the bacon into small pieces and put into the soup.
5. Cook on for about 30 minutes on low heat.
6. Season with salt and pepper and serve.

NUTRITION: Calories: 185 Carbs: 5.8g Fats: 12.7g Proteins: 10.8g Sodium: 1153mg Sugar: 2.4g

128. **Swiss Chard Egg Drop Soup**

Servings: 4

Preparation time: 20 mins

INGREDIENTS

- 3 cups bone broth
- 2 eggs, whisked
- 1 teaspoon ground oregano
- 3 tablespoons butter
- 2 cups Swiss chard, chopped
- 2 tablespoons coconut aminos
- 1 teaspoon ginger, grated
- Salt and black pepper, to taste

DIRECTIONS

1. Heat the bone broth in a saucepan and add whisked eggs while stirring slowly.
2. Add the swiss chard, butter, coconut aminos, ginger, oregano and salt and black pepper.
3. Cook for about 10 minutes and serve hot.

NUTRITION: Calories: 185 Carbs: 2.9g Fats: 11g Proteins: 18.3g Sodium: 252mg Sugar: 0.4g

129. Mushroom Spinach Soup

Servings: 4

Preparation time: 25 mins

INGREDIENTS

- 1cupspinach,cleaned and chopped
- 100gmushrooms,chopped
- 1onion
- 6 garlic cloves
- ½ teaspoon red chili powder
- Salt and black pepper, to taste
- 3 tablespoons buttermilk
- 1 teaspoon almond flour
- 2 cups chicken broth
- 3 tablespoons butter
- ¼ cup fresh cream,for garnish

DIRECTIONS

1. Heat butter in a pan and add onions and garlic.
2. Sauté for about 3 minutes and add spinach, salt and red chili powder.
3. Sauté for about 4 minutes and add mushrooms.

4. Transfer into a blender and blend to make a puree.
5. Return to the pan and add buttermilk and almond flour for creamy texture.
6. Mix well and simmer for about 2 minutes.
7. Garnish with fresh cream and serve hot.

NUTRITION: Calories: 160 Carbs: 7g Fats: 13.3g Proteins: 4.7g Sodium: 462mg Sugar: 2.7g

130. Delicata Squash Soup

Servings: 5

Preparation time: 45mins

Ingredients

- 1½ cups beef bone broth
- 1small onion, peeled and grated.
- ½ teaspoon sea salt
- ¼ teaspoon poultry seasoning
- 2small Delicata Squash, chopped
- 2 garlic cloves, minced
- 2tablespoons olive oil
- ¼ teaspoon black pepper
- 1 small lemon, juiced
- 5 tablespoons sour cream

DIRECTIONS

1. Put Delicata Squash and water in a medium pan and bring to a boil.
2. Reduce the heat and cook for about 20 minutes.
3. Drain and set aside.
4. Put olive oil, onions, garlic and poultry seasoning in a small sauce pan.
5. Cook for about 2 minutes and add broth.

6. Allow it to simmer for 5 minutes and remove from heat.
7. Whisk in the lemon juice and transfer the mixture in a blender.
8. Pulse until smooth and top with sour cream.

NUTRITION: Calories: 109 Carbs: 4.9g Fats: 8.5g Proteins: 3g Sodium: 279mg Sugar: 2.4g

131. Broccoli Soup

Servings: 6

Preparation time: 10 mins

INGREDIENTS

- 3 tablespoons ghee
- 5 garlic cloves
- 1 teaspoon sage
- ¼ teaspoon ginger
- 2 cups broccoli
- 1 small onion
- 1 teaspoon oregano
- ½ teaspoon parsley
- Salt and black pepper, to taste
- 6 cups vegetable broth
- 4 tablespoons butter

DIRECTIONS

1. Put ghee, onions, spices and garlic in a pot and cook for 3 minutes.
2. Add broccoli and cook for about 4 minutes.
3. Add vegetable broth, cover and allow it to simmer for about 30 minutes.
4. Transfer into a blender and blend until smooth.
5. Add the butter to give it a creamy delicious texture and flavor

NUTRITION: Calories: 183 Carbs: 5.2g Fats: 15.6g Proteins: 6.1g Sodium: 829mg Sugar: 1.8g

132. Apple Pumpkin Soup

Servings: 8

Preparation time: 10 mins

INGREDIENTS

- 1 apple, chopped
- 1 whole kabocha pumpkin, peeled, seeded and cubed
- 1 cup almond flour
- ¼ cup ghee
- 1 pinch cardamom powder
- 2 quarts water
- ¼ cup coconut cream
- 1 pinch ground black pepper

DIRECTIONS

1. Heat ghee in the bottom of a heavy pot and add apples.
2. Cook for about 5 minutes on a medium flame and add pumpkin.
3. Sauté for about 3 minutes and add almond flour.
4. Sauté for about 1 minute and add water.
5. Lower the flame and cook for about 30 minutes.
6. Transfer the soup into an immersion blender and blend until smooth.
7. Top with coconut cream and serve.

NUTRITION: Calories: 186 Carbs: 10.4g Fats: 14.9g Proteins: 3.7g Sodium: 7mg Sugar: 5.4g

133. Keto French Onion Soup

Servings: 6

Preparation time: 40 mins

INGREDIENTS

- 5 tablespoons butter
- 500 g brown onion medium
- 4 drops liquid stevia
- 4 tablespoons olive oil
- 3 cups beef stock

DIRECTIONS

1. Put the butter and olive oil in a large pot over medium low heat and add onions and salt.
2. Cook for about 5 minutes and stir in stevia.
3. Cook for another 5 minutes and add beef stock.
4. Reduce the heat to low and simmer for about 25 minutes.
5. Dish out into soup bowls and serve hot.

NUTRITION: Calories: 198 Carbs: 6g Fats: 20.6g Proteins: 2.9g Sodium: 883mg Sugar: 1.7g

134. Cauliflower and Thyme Soup

Servings: 6

Preparation time: 30 mins

INGREDIENTS

- 2teaspoonsthyme powder
- 1head cauliflower
- 3cupsvegetable stock

- ½ teaspoon matcha green tea powder
- 3tablespoonsolive oil
- Salt and black pepper, to taste
- 5garlic cloves,chopped

DIRECTIONS

1. Put the vegetable stock, thyme and matcha powder to a large pot over medium-high heat and bring to a boil.
2. Add cauliflower and cook for about 10 minutes.
3. Meanwhile, put the olive oil and garlic in a small sauce pan and cook for about 1 minute.
4. Add the garlic, salt and black pepper and cook for about 2 minutes.
5. Transfer into an immersion blender and blend until smooth.
6. Dish out and serve immediately.

NUTRITION: Calories: 79 Carbs: 3.8g Fats: 7.1g Proteins: 1.3g Sodium: 39mg Sugar: 1.5g

135. Homemade Thai Chicken Soup

Servings: 12

Preparation time: 8 hours 25 mins

Ingredients

- 1 lemongrass stalk, cut into large chunks
- 5 thick slices of fresh ginger
- 1 whole chicken
- 20 fresh basil leaves
- 1 lime, juiced
- 1 tablespoon salt

DIRECTIONS

1. Place the chicken, 10 basil leaves, lemongrass, ginger, salt and water into the slow cooker.
2. Cook for about 8 hours on low and dish out into a bowl.
3. Stir in fresh lime juice and basil leaves to serve.

NUTRITION: Calories: 255 Carbs: 1.2g Fats: 17.6g Proteins: 25.2g Sodium: 582mg Sugar: 0.1g

136. Chicken Kale Soup

Servings: 6

Preparation time: 6 hours 10 mins

INGREDIENTS

- 2poundschicken breast, skinless
- 1/3cuponion
- 1tablespoonolive oil
- 14ounceschicken bone broth
- ½ cup olive oil
- 4 cups chicken stock
- ¼ cup lemon juice
- 5ouncesbaby kale leaves
- Salt, to taste

DIRECTIONS

1. Season chicken with salt and black pepper.
2. Heat olive oil over medium heat in a large skillet and add seasoned chicken.
3. Reduce the temperature and cook for about 15 minutes.
4. Shred the chicken and place in the crock pot.

5. Process the chicken broth and onions in a blender and blend until smooth.
6. Pour into crock pot and stir in the remaining ingredients.
7. Cook on low for about 6 hours, stirring once while cooking.

NUTRITION: Calories: 261 Carbs: 2g Fats: 21g Proteins: 14.1g Sodium: 264mg Sugar: 0.3g

137. Chicken Veggie Soup

Servings: 6

Preparation time: 20 mins

INGREDIENTS

- 5 chicken thighs
- 12 cups water
- 1 tablespoon adobo seasoning
- 4 celery ribs
- 1 yellow onion
- 1½ teaspoons whole black peppercorns
- 6 sprigs fresh parsley
- 2 teaspoons coarse sea salt
- 2 carrots
- 6 mushrooms, sliced
- 2 garlic cloves
- 1 bay leaf
- 3 sprigs fresh thyme

DIRECTIONS

1. Put water, chicken thighs, carrots, celery ribs, onion, garlic cloves and herbs in a large pot.
2. Bring to a boil and reduce the heat to low.
3. Cover the pot and simmer for about 30 minutes.

4. Dish out the chicken and shred it, removing the bones.
5. Put the bones back into the pot and simmer for about 20 minutes.
6. Strain the broth, discarding the chunks and put the liquid back into the pot.
7. Bring it to a boil and simmer for about 30 minutes.
8. Put the mushrooms in the broth and simmer for about 10 minutes.
9. Dish out to serve hot.

NUTRITION: Calories: 250 Carbs: 6.4g Fats: 8.9g Proteins: 35.1g Sodium: 852mg Sugar: 2.5g

138. **Chicken Mulligatawny Soup**

Servings: 10

Preparation time: 30 mins

INGREDIENTS

- 1½ tablespoons curry powder
- 3 cups celery root, diced
- 2 tablespoons Swerve
- 10 cups chicken broth
- 5 cups chicken, chopped and cooked
- ¼ cup apple cider
- ½ cup sour cream
- ¼ cup fresh parsley, chopped
- 2 tablespoons butter
- Salt and black pepper, to taste

DIRECTIONS

1. Combine the broth, butter, chicken, curry powder, celery root and apple cider in a large soup pot.
2. Bring to a boil and simmer for about 30 minutes.

3. Stir in Swerve, sour cream, fresh parsley, salt and black pepper.
4. Dish out and serve hot.

NUTRITION: Calories: 215 Carbs: 7.1g Fats: 8.5g Proteins: 26.4g Sodium: 878mg Sugar: 2.2g

139. **Buffalo Ranch Chicken Soup**

Servings: 4

Preparation time: 40 mins

INGREDIENTS

- 2 tablespoons parsley
- 2 celery stalks, chopped
- 6 tablespoons butter
- 1 cup heavy whipping cream
- 4 cups chicken, cooked and shredded
- 4 tablespoons ranch dressing
- ¼ cup yellow onions, chopped
- 8 oz cream cheese
- 8 cups chicken broth
- 7 hearty bacon slices, crumbled

DIRECTIONS

1. Heat butter in a pan and add chicken.
2. Cook for about 5 minutes and add 1½ cups water.
3. Cover and cook for about 10 minutes.
4. Put the chicken and rest of the ingredients into the saucepan except parsley and cook for about 10 minutes.
5. Top with parsley and serve hot.

NUTRITION: Calories: 444 Carbs: 4g Fats: 34g Proteins: 28g Sodium: 1572mg Sugar: 2g

140. **Traditional Chicken Soup**

Servings: 6

Preparation time: 1 hour 45 mins

INGREDIENTS

- 3 pounds chicken
- 4 quarts water
- 4 stalks celery
- 1/3 large red onion
- 1 large carrot
- 3 garlic cloves
- 2 thyme sprigs
- 2 rosemary sprigs
- Salt and black pepper, to taste

DIRECTIONS

1. Put water and chicken in the stock pot on medium high heat.
2. Bring to a boil and allow it to simmer for about 10 minutes.
3. Add onion, garlic, celery, salt and pepper and simmer on medium low heat for 30 minutes.
4. Add thyme and carrots and simmer on low for another 30 minutes.
5. Dish out the chicken and shred the pieces, removing the bones.
6. Return the chicken pieces to the pot and add rosemary sprigs.
7. Simmer for about 20 minutes at low heat and dish out to serve.

NUTRITION: Calories: 357 Carbs: 3.3g Fats: 7g Proteins: 66.2g Sodium: 175mg Sugar: 1.1g

141. **Chicken Noodle Soup**

Servings: 6

Preparation time: 30 mins

INGREDIENTS

- 1 onion, minced
- 1 rib celery, sliced
- 3 cups chicken, shredded
- 3 eggs, lightly beaten
- 1 green onion, for garnish
- 2 tablespoons coconut oil
- 1 carrot, peeled and thinly sliced
- 2 teaspoons dried thyme
- 2½ quarts homemade bone broth
- ¼ cup fresh parsley, minced
- Salt and black pepper, to taste

DIRECTIONS

1. Heat coconut oil over medium-high heat in a large pot and add onions, carrots, and celery.
2. Cook for about 4 minutes and stir in the bone broth, thyme and chicken.
3. Simmer for about 15 minutes and stir in parsley.
4. Pour beaten eggs into the soup in a slow steady stream.
5. Remove soup from heat and let it stand for about 2 minutes.
6. Season with salt and black pepper and dish out to serve.

NUTRITION: Calories: 226 Carbs: 3.5g Fats: 8.9g Proteins: 31.8g Sodium: 152mg Sugar: 1.6g

142. **Chicken Cabbage Soup**

Servings: 8

Preparation time: 35 mins

INGREDIENTS

- 2celery stalks
- 2garlic cloves, minced
- 4 oz.butter
- 6 oz. mushrooms, sliced
- 2 tablespoons onions, dried and minced
- 1 teaspoon salt
- 8 cups chicken broth
- 1medium carrot
- 2 cups green cabbage, sliced into strips
- 2 teaspoons dried parsley
- ¼ teaspoon black pepper
- 1½ rotisserie chickens, shredded

DIRECTIONS

1. Melt butter in a large pot and add celery, mushrooms, onions and garlic into the pot.
2. Cook for about 4 minutes and add broth, parsley, carrot, salt and black pepper.
3. Simmer for about 10 minutes and add cooked chicken and cabbage.
4. Simmer for an additional 12 minutes until the cabbage is tender.
5. Dish out and serve hot.

NUTRITION: Calories: 184 Carbs: 4.2g Fats: 13.1g Proteins: 12.6g Sodium: 1244mg Sugar: 2.1g

143. Green Chicken Enchilada Soup

Servings: 5

Preparation time: 20 mins

INGREDIENTS

- 4 oz. cream cheese, softened
- ½ cup salsa verde
- 1 cup cheddar cheese, shredded
- 2 cups cooked chicken, shredded
- 2 cups chicken stock

DIRECTIONS

1. Put salsa verde, cheddar cheese, cream cheese and chicken stock in an immersion blender and blend until smooth.
2. Pour this mixture into a medium saucepan and cook for about 5 minutes on medium heat.
3. Add the shredded chicken and cook for about 5 minutes.
4. Garnish with additional shredded cheddar and serve hot.

NUTRITION: Calories: 265 Carbs: 2.2g Fats: 17.4g Proteins: 24.2g Sodium: 686mg Sugar: 0.8g

144. Keto BBQ Chicken Pizza Soup

Servings: 6

Preparation time: 1 hour 30 mins

INGREDIENTS

- 6 chicken legs
- 1 medium red onion, diced
- 4 garlic cloves
- 1 large tomato, unsweetened
- 4 cups green beans
- ¾ cup BBQ Sauce
- 1½ cups mozzarella cheese, shredded
- ¼ cup ghee

- 2 quarts water
- 2 quarts chicken stock
- Salt and black pepper, to taste
- Fresh cilantro, for garnishing

DIRECTIONS

1. Put chicken, water and salt in a large pot and bring to a boil.
2. Reduce the heat to medium-low and cook for about 75 minutes.
3. Shred the meat off the bones using a fork and keep aside.
4. Put ghee, red onions and garlic in a large soup and cook over a medium heat.
5. Add chicken stock and bring to a boil over a high heat.
6. Add green beans and tomato to the pot and cook for about 15 minutes.
7. AddBBQ Sauce, shredded chicken, salt and black pepper to the pot.
8. Ladle the soup into serving bowls and top with shredded mozzarella cheese and cilantro to serve.

NUTRITION: Calories: 449 Carbs: 7.1g Fats: 32.5g Proteins: 30.8g Sodium: 252mg Sugar: 4.7g

145. Salmon Stew Soup

Servings: 5

Preparation time: 25 mins

INGREDIENTS

- 4 cups chicken broth
- 3 salmon fillets, chunked
- 2 tablespoons butter
- 1 cup parsley, chopped
- 3 cups Swiss chard, roughly chopped
- 2 Italian squash, chopped

- 1 garlic clove, crushed
- ½ lemon, juiced
- Salt and black pepper, to taste
- 2 eggs

DIRECTIONS

1. Put the chicken broth and garlic into a pot and bring to a boil.
2. Add salmon, lemon juice and butter in the pot and cook for about 10 minutes on medium heat.
3. Add Swiss chard, Italian squash, salt and pepper and cook for about 10 minutes.
4. Whisk eggs and add to the pot, stirring continuously.
5. Garnish with parsley and serve.

NUTRITION: Calories: 262 Carbs: 7.8g Fats: 14g Proteins: 27.5g Sodium: 1021mg Sugar: 1.2g

146. Spicy Halibut Tomato Soup

Servings: 8

Preparation time: 1 hour 5mins

INGREDIENTS

- 2garliccloves, minced
- 1tablespoonolive oil
- ¼ cup fresh parsley, chopped
- 10anchoviescanned in oil, minced
- 6cupsvegetable broth
- 1teaspoonblack pepper
- 1poundhalibut fillets, chopped
- 3tomatoes, peeled and diced
- 1teaspoonsalt
- 1teaspoonred chili flakes

DIRECTIONS

1. Heat olive oil in a large stockpot over medium heat and add garlic and half of the parsley.
2. Add anchovies, tomatoes, vegetable broth, red chili flakes, salt and black pepper and bring to a boil.
3. Reduce the heat to medium-low and simmer for about 20 minutes.
4. Add halibut fillets and cook for about 10 minutes.
5. Dish out the halibut and shred into small pieces.
6. Mix back with the soup and garnish with the remaining fresh parsley to serve.

NUTRITION: Calories: 170 Carbs: 3g Fats: 6.7g Proteins: 23.4g Sodium: 2103mg Sugar: 1.8g

PASTA, RICE & GRAINS

147. Delicious Chicken Pasta

Preparation Time: 10 minutes

Cooking Time: 17 minutes

Servings: 4

INGREDIENTS

- 3 chicken breasts, skinless, boneless, cut into pieces
- 9 oz whole-grain pasta
- 1/2 cup olives, sliced
- 1/2 cup sun-dried tomatoes
- 1 tbsp roasted red peppers, chopped
- 14 oz can tomatoes, diced
- 2 cups marinara sauce
- 1 cup chicken broth
- Pepper
- Salt

DIRECTIONS

1. Add all ingredients except whole-grain pasta into the instant pot and stir well.
2. Seal pot with lid and cook on high for 12 minutes.
3. Once done, allow to release pressure naturally. Remove lid.
4. Add pasta and stir well. Seal pot again and select manual and set timer for 5 minutes.
5. Once done, allow to release pressure naturally for 5 minutes then release remaining using quick release. Remove lid.
6. Stir well and serve.

NUTRITION: Calories 615 Fat 15.4 g Carbohydrates 71 g Sugar 17.6 g Protein 48 g Cholesterol 100 mg

148. Flavors Taco Rice Bowl

Preparation Time: 10 minutes

Cooking Time: 14 minutes

Servings: 8

INGREDIENTS

- 1 lb ground beef
- 8 oz cheddar cheese, shredded
- 14 oz can red beans
- 2 oz taco seasoning
- 16 oz salsa
- 2 cups of water
- 2 cups brown rice
- Pepper
- Salt

DIRECTIONS

1. Set instant pot on sauté mode.
2. Add meat to the pot and sauté until brown.
3. Add water, beans, rice, taco seasoning, pepper, and salt and stir well.
4. Top with salsa. Seal pot with lid and cook on high for 14 minutes.
5. Once done, release pressure using quick release. Remove lid.
6. Add cheddar cheese and stir until cheese is melted.
7. Serve and enjoy.

NUTRITION: Calories 464 Fat 15.3 g Carbohydrates 48.9 g Sugar 2.8 g Protein 32.2 g Cholesterol 83 mg

149. <u>Flavorful Mac & Cheese</u>

Preparation Time: 10 minutes

Cooking Time: 10 minutes

Servings: 6

INGREDIENTS

- 16 oz whole-grain elbow pasta
- 4 cups of water
- 1 cup can tomatoes, diced
- 1 tsp garlic, chopped
- 2 tbsp olive oil
- 1/4 cup green onions, chopped
- 1/2 cup parmesan cheese, grated
- 1/2 cup mozzarella cheese, grated
- 1 cup cheddar cheese, grated
- 1/4 cup passata
- 1 cup unsweetened almond milk
- 1 cup marinated artichoke, diced
- 1/2 cup sun-dried tomatoes, sliced
- 1/2 cup olives, sliced
- 1 tsp salt

DIRECTIONS

1. Add pasta, water, tomatoes, garlic, oil, and salt into the instant pot and stir well.
2. Seal pot with lid and cook on high for 4 minutes.
3. Once done, allow to release pressure naturally for 5 minutes then release remaining using quick release. Remove lid.
4. Set pot on sauté mode. Add green onion, parmesan cheese, mozzarella cheese, cheddar cheese, passata, almond milk, artichoke, sun-dried tomatoes, and olive. Mix well.
5. Stir well and cook until cheese is melted.
6. Serve and enjoy.

NUTRITION: Calories 519 Fat 17.1 g Carbohydrates 66.5 g Sugar 5.2 g Protein 25 g Cholesterol 26 mg

150. <u>Cucumber Olive Rice</u>

Preparation Time: 10 minutes

Cooking Time: 10 minutes

Servings: 8

INGREDIENTS

- 2 cups rice, rinsed
- 1/2 cup olives, pitted
- 1 cup cucumber, chopped
- 1 tbsp red wine vinegar
- 1 tsp lemon zest, grated
- 1 tbsp fresh lemon juice
- 2 tbsp olive oil
- 2 cups vegetable broth
- 1/2 tsp dried oregano
- 1 red bell pepper, chopped
- 1/2 cup onion, chopped
- 1 tbsp olive oil
- Pepper
- Salt

DIRECTIONS

1. Add oil into the inner pot of instant pot and set the pot on sauté mode.
2. Add onion and sauté for 3 minutes.
3. Add bell pepper and oregano and sauté for 1 minute.
4. Add rice and broth and stir well.

5. Seal pot with lid and cook on high for 6 minutes.
6. Once done, allow to release pressure naturally for 10 minutes then release remaining using quick release. Remove lid.
7. Add remaining ingredients and stir everything well to mix.
8. Serve immediately and enjoy it.

NUTRITION: Calories 229 Fat 5.1 g Carbohydrates 40.2 g Sugar 1.6 g Protein 4.9 g Cholesterol 0 mg

151. **Flavors Herb Risotto**

Preparation Time: 10 minutes

Cooking Time: 15 minutes

Servings: 4

INGREDIENTS

- 2 cups of rice
- 2 tbsp parmesan cheese, grated
- 3.5 oz heavy cream
- 1 tbsp fresh oregano, chopped
- 1 tbsp fresh basil, chopped
- 1/2 tbsp sage, chopped
- 1 onion, chopped
- 2 tbsp olive oil
- 1 tsp garlic, minced
- 4 cups vegetable stock
- Pepper
- Salt

DIRECTIONS

1. Add oil into the inner pot of instant pot and set the pot on sauté mode.
2. Add garlic and onion and sauté for 2-3 minutes.

3. Add remaining ingredients except for parmesan cheese and heavy cream and stir well.
4. Seal pot with lid and cook on high for 12 minutes.
5. Once done, allow to release pressure naturally for 10 minutes then release remaining using quick release. Remove lid.
6. Stir in cream and cheese and serve.

NUTRITION: Calories 514 Fat 17.6 g Carbohydrates 79.4 g Sugar 2.1 g Protein 8.8 g Cholesterol 36 mg

152. **Delicious Pasta Primavera**

Preparation Time: 10 minutes

Cooking Time: 4 minutes

Servings: 4

INGREDIENTS

- 8 oz whole wheat penne pasta
- 1 tbsp fresh lemon juice
- 2 tbsp fresh parsley, chopped
- 1/4 cup almonds slivered
- 1/4 cup parmesan cheese, grated
- 14 oz can tomatoes, diced
- 1/2 cup prunes
- 1/2 cup zucchini, chopped
- 1/2 cup asparagus, cut into 1-inch pieces
- 1/2 cup carrots, chopped
- 1/2 cup broccoli, chopped
- 1 3/4 cups vegetable stock
- Pepper
- Salt

DIRECTIONS

1. Add stock, pars, tomatoes, prunes, zucchini, asparagus, carrots, and broccoli into the instant pot and stir well.
2. Seal pot with lid and cook on high for 4 minutes.
3. Once done, release pressure using quick release. Remove lid.
4. Add remaining ingredients and stir well and serve.

NUTRITION: Calories 303 Fat 2.6 g Carbohydrates 63.5 g Sugar 13.4 g Protein 12.8 g Cholesterol 1 mg

153. Roasted Pepper Pasta

Preparation Time: 10 minutes

Cooking Time: 13 minutes

Servings: 6

INGREDIENTS

- 1 lb whole wheat penne pasta
- 1 tbsp Italian seasoning
- 4 cups vegetable broth
- 1 tbsp garlic, minced
- 1/2 onion, chopped
- 14 oz jar roasted red peppers
- 1 cup feta cheese, crumbled
- 1 tbsp olive oil
- Pepper
- Salt

DIRECTIONS

1. Add roasted pepper into the blender and blend until smooth.
2. Add oil into the inner pot of instant pot and set the pot on sauté mode.

3. Add garlic and onion and sauté for 2-3 minutes.
4. Add blended roasted pepper and sauté for 2 minutes.
5. Add remaining ingredients except feta cheese and stir well.
6. Seal pot with lid and cook on high for 8 minutes.
7. Once done, allow to release pressure naturally for 5 minutes then release remaining using quick release. Remove lid.
8. Top with feta cheese and serve.

NUTRITION: Calories 459 Fat 10.6 g Carbohydrates 68.1 g Sugar 2.1 g Protein 21.3 g Cholesterol 24 mg

154. Cheese Basil Tomato Rice

Preparation Time: 10 minutes

Cooking Time: 26 minutes

Servings: 8

INGREDIENTS

- 1 1/2 cups brown rice
- 1 cup parmesan cheese, grated
- 1/4 cup fresh basil, chopped
- 2 cups grape tomatoes, halved
- 8 oz can tomato sauce
- 1 3/4 cup vegetable broth
- 1 tbsp garlic, minced
- 1/2 cup onion, diced
- 1 tbsp olive oil
- Pepper
- Salt

DIRECTIONS

1. Add oil into the inner pot of instant pot and set the pot on sauté mode.

2. Add garlic and onion and sauté for 4 minutes.
3. Add rice, tomato sauce, broth, pepper, and salt and stir well.
4. Seal pot with lid and cook on high for 22 minutes.
5. Once done, allow to release pressure naturally for 10 minutes then release remaining using quick release. Remove lid.
6. Add remaining ingredients and stir well.
7. Serve and enjoy.

NUTRITION: Calories 208 Fat 5.6 g Carbohydrates 32.1 g Sugar 2.8 g Protein 8.3 g Cholesterol 8 mg

155. Mac & Cheese

Preparation Time: 10 minutes

Cooking Time: 4 minutes

Servings: 8

INGREDIENTS

- 1 lb whole grain pasta
- 1/2 cup parmesan cheese, grated
- 4 cups cheddar cheese, shredded
- 1 cup milk
- 1/4 tsp garlic powder
- 1/2 tsp ground mustard
- 2 tbsp olive oil
- 4 cups of water
- Pepper
- Salt

DIRECTIONS

1. Add pasta, garlic powder, mustard, oil, water, pepper, and salt into the instant pot.

2. Seal pot with lid and cook on high for 4 minutes.
3. Once done, release pressure using quick release. Remove lid.
4. Add remaining ingredients and stir well and serve.

NUTRITION: Calories 509 Fat 25.7 g Carbohydrates 43.8 g Sugar 3.8 g Protein 27.3 g Cholesterol 66 mg

156. Tuna Pasta

Preparation Time: 10 minutes

Cooking Time: 8 minutes

Servings: 6

INGREDIENTS

- 10 oz can tuna, drained
- 15 oz whole wheat rotini pasta
- 4 oz mozzarella cheese, cubed
- 1/2 cup parmesan cheese, grated
- 1 tsp dried basil
- 14 oz can tomatoes, diced
- 4 cups vegetable broth
- 1 tbsp garlic, minced
- 8 oz mushrooms, sliced
- 2 zucchini, sliced
- 1 onion, chopped
- 2 tbsp olive oil
- Pepper
- Salt

DIRECTIONS

1. Add oil into the inner pot of instant pot and set the pot on sauté mode.
2. Add mushrooms, zucchini, and onion and sauté until onion is softened.
3. Add garlic and sauté for a minute.

4. Add pasta, basil, tuna, tomatoes, and broth and stir well.
5. Seal pot with lid and cook on high for 4 minutes.
6. Once done, allow to release pressure naturally for 5 minutes then release remaining using quick release. Remove lid.
7. Add remaining ingredients and stir well and serve.

NUTRITION: Calories 346 Fat 11.9 g Carbohydrates 31.3 g Sugar 6.3 g Protein 6.3 g Cholesterol 30 mg

157. Vegan Olive Pasta

Preparation Time: 10 minutes

Cooking Time: 5 minutes

Servings: 4

INGREDIENTS

- 4 cups whole grain penne pasta
- 1/2 cup olives, sliced
- 1 tbsp capers
- 1/4 tsp red pepper flakes
- 3 cups of water
- 4 cups pasta sauce, homemade
- 1 tbsp garlic, minced
- Pepper
- Salt

DIRECTIONS

1. Add all ingredients into the inner pot of instant pot and stir well.
2. Seal pot with lid and cook on high for 5 minutes.
3. Once done, release pressure using quick release. Remove lid.
4. Stir and serve.

NUTRITION: Calories 441 Fat 10.1 g Carbohydrates 77.3 g Sugar 24.1 g Protein 11.8 g Cholesterol 5 mg

158. Italian Mac & Cheese

Preparation Time: 10 minutes

Cooking Time: 6 minutes

Servings: 4

INGREDIENTS

- 1 lb whole grain pasta
- 2 tsp Italian seasoning
- 1 1/2 tsp garlic powder
- 1 1/2 tsp onion powder
- 1 cup sour cream
- 4 cups of water
- 4 oz parmesan cheese, shredded
- 12 oz ricotta cheese
- Pepper
- Salt

DIRECTIONS

1. Add all ingredients except ricotta cheese into the inner pot of instant pot and stir well.
2. Seal pot with lid and cook on high for 6 minutes.
3. Once done, allow to release pressure naturally for 5 minutes then release remaining using quick release. Remove lid.
4. Add ricotta cheese and stir well and serve.

NUTRITION Calories 388 Fat 25.8 g Carbohydrates 18.1 g Sugar 4 g Protein 22.8 g Cholesterol 74 mg

159. Italian Chicken Pasta

Preparation Time: 10 minutes

Cooking Time: 9 minutes

Servings: 8

INGREDIENTS

- 1 lb chicken breast, skinless, boneless, and cut into chunks
- 1/2 cup cream cheese
- 1 cup mozzarella cheese, shredded
- 1 1/2 tsp Italian seasoning
- 1 tsp garlic, minced
- 1 cup mushrooms, diced
- 1/2 onion, diced
- 2 tomatoes, diced
- 2 cups of water
- 16 oz whole wheat penne pasta
- Pepper
- Salt

DIRECTIONS

1. Add all ingredients except cheeses into the inner pot of instant pot and stir well.
2. Seal pot with lid and cook on high for 9 minutes.
3. Once done, allow to release pressure naturally for 5 minutes then release remaining using quick release. Remove lid.
4. Add cheeses and stir well and serve.

NUTRITION: Calories 328 Fat 8.5 g Carbohydrates 42.7 g Sugar 1.4 g Protein 23.7 g Cholesterol 55 mg

160. Delicious Greek Chicken Pasta

Preparation Time: 10 minutes

Cooking Time: 10 minutes

Servings: 6

INGREDIENTS

- 2 chicken breasts, skinless, boneless, and cut into chunks
- 1/2 cup olives, sliced
- 2 cups vegetable stock
- 12 oz Greek vinaigrette dressing
- 1 lb whole grain pasta
- Pepper
- Salt

DIRECTIONS

1. Add all ingredients into the inner pot of instant pot and stir well.
2. Seal pot with lid and cook on high for 10 minutes.
3. Once done, release pressure using quick release. Remove lid.
4. Stir well and serve.

NUTRITION: Calories 325 Fat 25.8 g Carbohydrates 10.5 g Sugar 4 g Protein 15.6 g Cholesterol 43 mg

161. Pesto Chicken Pasta

Preparation Time: 10 minutes

Cooking Time: 10 minutes

Servings: 6

INGREDIENTS

- 1 lb chicken breast, skinless, boneless, and diced
- 3 tbsp olive oil
- 1/2 cup parmesan cheese, shredded
- 1 tsp Italian seasoning
- 1/4 cup heavy cream
- 16 oz whole wheat pasta
- 6 oz basil pesto
- 3 1/2 cups water
- Pepper
- Salt

DIRECTIONS

1. Season chicken with Italian seasoning, pepper, and salt.
2. Add oil into the inner pot of instant pot and set the pot on sauté mode.
3. Add chicken to the pot and sauté until brown.
4. Add remaining ingredients except for parmesan cheese, heavy cream, and pesto and stir well.
5. Seal pot with lid and cook on high for 5 minutes.
6. Once done, release pressure using quick release. Remove lid.
7. Stir in parmesan cheese, heavy cream, and pesto and serve.

NUTRITION: Calories 475 Fat 14.7 g Carbohydrates 57 g Sugar 2.8 g Protein 28.7 g Cholesterol 61 mg

162. Spinach Pesto Pasta

Preparation Time: 10 minutes

Cooking Time: 10 minutes

Servings: 4

INGREDIENTS

- 8 oz whole-grain pasta
- 1/3 cup mozzarella cheese, grated
- 1/2 cup pesto
- 5 oz fresh spinach
- 1 3/4 cup water
- 8 oz mushrooms, chopped
- 1 tbsp olive oil
- Pepper
- Salt

DIRECTIONS

1. Add oil into the inner pot of instant pot and set the pot on sauté mode.
2. Add mushrooms and sauté for 5 minutes.
3. Add water and pasta and stir well.
4. Seal pot with lid and cook on high for 5 minutes.
5. Once done, release pressure using quick release. Remove lid.
6. Stir in remaining ingredients and serve.

NUTRITION: Calories 213 Fat 17.3 g Carbohydrates 9.5 g Sugar 4.5 g Protein 7.4 g Cholesterol 9 mg

163. Fiber Packed Chicken Rice

Preparation Time: 10 minutes

Cooking Time: 16 minutes

Servings: 6

INGREDIENTS

- 1 lb chicken breast, skinless, boneless, and cut into chunks
- 14.5 oz can cannellini beans

- 4 cups chicken broth
- 2 cups wild rice
- 1 tbsp Italian seasoning
- 1 small onion, chopped
- 1 tbsp garlic, chopped
- 1 tbsp olive oil
- Pepper
- Salt

DIRECTIONS

- Add oil into the inner pot of instant pot and set the pot on sauté mode.
- Add garlic and onion and sauté for 2 minutes.
- Add chicken and cook for 2 minutes.
- Add remaining ingredients and stir well.
- Seal pot with lid and cook on high for 12 minutes.
- Once done, release pressure using quick release. Remove lid.
- Stir well and serve.

NUTRITION: Calories 399 Fat 6.4 g Carbohydrates 53.4 g Sugar 3 g Protein 31.6 g Cholesterol 50 mg

164. Tasty Greek Rice

Preparation Time: 10 minutes

Cooking Time: 10 minutes

Servings: 6

INGREDIENTS

- 1 3/4 cup brown rice, rinsed and drained
- 3/4 cup roasted red peppers, chopped
- 1 cup olives, chopped
- 1 tsp dried oregano

- 1 tsp Greek seasoning
- 1 3/4 cup vegetable broth
- 2 tbsp olive oil
- Salt

DIRECTIONS

1. Add oil into the inner pot of instant pot and set the pot on sauté mode.
2. Add rice and cook for 5 minutes.
3. Add remaining ingredients except for red peppers and olives and stir well.
4. Seal pot with lid and cook on high for 5 minutes.
5. Once done, allow to release pressure naturally for 10 minutes then release remaining using quick release. Remove lid.
6. Add red peppers and olives and stir well.
7. Serve and enjoy. Ingredients

NUTRITION: Calories 285 Fat 9.1 g Carbohydrates 45.7 g Sugar 1.2 g Protein 6 g Cholesterol 0 mg

165. Bulgur Salad

Preparation Time: 10 minutes

Cooking Time: 1 minute

Servings: 2

INGREDIENTS

- 1/2 cup bulgur wheat
- 1/4 cup fresh parsley, chopped
- 1 tbsp fresh mint, chopped
- 1/3 cup feta cheese, crumbled
- 2 tbsp fresh lemon juice
- 2 tbsp olives, chopped
- 1/4 cup olive oil
- 1/2 cup tomatoes, chopped

- 1/3 cup cucumber, chopped
- 1/2 cup water
- Salt

DIRECTIONS

1. Add the bulgur wheat, water, and salt into the instant pot.
2. Seal pot with lid and cook on high for 1 minute.
3. Once done, release pressure using quick release. Remove lid.
4. Transfer bulgur wheat to the mixing bowl. Add remaining ingredients to the bowl and mix well.
5. Serve and enjoy.

NUTRITION: Calories 430 Fat 32.2 g Carbohydrates 31.5 g Sugar 3 g Protein 8.9 g Cholesterol 22 mg

166. **Perfect Herb Rice**

Preparation Time: 10 minutes

Cooking Time: 4 minutes

Servings: 4

INGREDIENTS

- 1 cup brown rice, rinsed
- 1 tbsp olive oil
- 1 1/2 cups water
- 1/2 cup fresh mix herbs, chopped
- 1 tsp salt

DIRECTIONS

1. Add all ingredients into the inner pot of instant pot and stir well.
2. Seal pot with lid and cook on high for 4 minutes.

3. Once done, allow to release pressure naturally for 10 minutes then release remaining using quick release. Remove lid.
4. Stir well and serve.

NUTRITION: Calories 264 Fat 9.9 g Carbohydrates 36.7 g Sugar 0.4 g Protein 7.3 g Cholesterol 0 mg

167. **Herb Polenta**

Preparation Time: 10 minutes

Cooking Time: 12 minutes

Servings: 6

INGREDIENTS

- 1 cup polenta
- 1/4 tsp nutmeg
- 3 tbsp fresh parsley, chopped
- 1/4 cup milk
- 1/2 cup parmesan cheese, grated
- 4 cups vegetable broth
- 2 tsp thyme, chopped
- 2 tsp rosemary, chopped
- 2 tsp sage, chopped
- 1 small onion, chopped
- 2 tbsp olive oil
- Salt

DIRECTIONS

1. Add oil into the inner pot of instant pot and set the pot on sauté mode.
2. Add onion and herbs and sauté for 4 minutes.
3. Add polenta, broth, and salt and stir well.
4. Seal pot with lid and cook on high for 8 minutes.

5. Once done, allow to release pressure naturally. Remove lid.
6. Stir in remaining ingredients and serve.

NUTRITION: Calories 196 Fat 7.8 g Carbohydrates 23.5 g Sugar 1.7 g Protein 8.2 g Cholesterol 6 mg

168. <u>Pecorino Pasta with Sausage and Fresh Tomato</u>

Servings: 4,

Cooking Time: 20 minutes

INGREDIENTS

- ¼ cup torn fresh basil leaves
- 1/8 tsp black pepper
- ¼ tsp salt
- 6 tbsp grated fresh pecorino Romano cheese, divided
- 1 ¼ lbs. tomatoes, chopped
- 2 tsp minced garlic
- 1 cup vertically sliced onions
- 2 tsp olive oil
- 8 oz sweet Italian sausage
- 8 oz uncooked penne, cooked and drained

DIRECTIONS

1. On medium high fire, place a nonstick fry pan with oil and cook for five minutes onion and sausage. Stir constantly to break sausage into pieces.
2. Stir in garlic and continue cooking for two minutes more.
3. Add tomatoes and cook for another two minutes.
4. Remove pan from fire, season with pepper and salt. Mix well.

5. Stir in 2 tbsp cheese and pasta. Toss well.
6. Transfer to a serving dish, garnish with basil and remaining cheese before serving.

NUTRITION: Calories: 376; Carbs: 50.8g; Protein: 17.8g; Fat: 11.6g

169. <u>Pesto Pasta and Shrimps</u>

Servings: 4,

Cooking Time: 15 minutes

INGREDIENTS

- ¼ cup pesto, divided
- ¼ cup shaved Parmesan Cheese
- 1 ¼ lbs. large shrimp, peeled and deveined
- 1 cup halved grape tomatoes
- 4-oz angel hair pasta, cooked, rinsed and drained

DIRECTIONS

1. On medium high fire, place a nonstick large fry pan and grease with cooking spray.
2. Add tomatoes, pesto and shrimp. Cook for 15 minutes or until shrimps are opaque, while covered.
3. Stir in cooked pasta and cook until heated through.
4. Transfer to a serving plate and garnish with Parmesan cheese.

NUTRITION: Calories: 319; Carbs: 23.6g; Protein: 31.4g; Fat: 11g

170. <u>Prosciutto e Faggioli</u>

Servings: 4,

Cooking Time: 15 minutes

INGREDIENTS

- 12 oz pasta, cooked and drained
- Pepper and salt to taste
- 3 tbsp snipped fresh chives
- 3 cups arugula or watercress leaves, loosely packed
- ½ cup chicken broth, warm
- 1 tbsp Herbed garlic butter
- ½ cup shredded pecorino Toscano
- 4 oz prosciutto, cut into bite sizes
- 2 cups cherry tomatoes, halved
- 1 can of 19oz white kidney beans, rinsed and drained

DIRECTIONS

1. Heat over medium low fire herbed garlic butter, cheese, prosciutto, tomatoes and beans in a big saucepan for 2 minutes.
2. Once mixture is simmering, stir constantly to melt cheese while gradually stirring in the broth.
3. Once cheese is fully melted and incorporated, add chives, arugula, pepper and salt.
4. Turn off the fire and toss in the cooked pasta. Serve and enjoy.

NUTRITION: Calories: 452; Carbs: 57.9g; Protein: 30.64g; Fat: 11.7g

171. **Puttanesca Style Bucatini**

Servings: 4,

Cooking Time: 40 minutes

INGREDIENTS

- 1 tbsp capers, rinsed

- 1 tsp coarsely chopped fresh oregano
- 1 tsp finely chopped garlic
- 1/8 tsp salt
- 12-oz bucatini pasta
- 2 cups coarsely chopped canned no-salt-added whole peeled tomatoes with their juice
- 3 tbsp extra virgin olive oil, divided
- 4 anchovy fillets, chopped
- 8 black Kalamata olives, pitted and sliced into slivers

DIRECTIONS

1. Cook bucatini pasta according to package directions. Drain, keep warm, and set aside.
2. On medium fire, place a large nonstick saucepan and heat 2 tbsp oil.
3. Sauté anchovies until it starts to disintegrate.
4. Add garlic and sauté for 15 seconds.
5. Add tomatoes, sauté for 15 to 20 minutes or until no longer watery. Season with 1/8 tsp salt.
6. Add oregano, capers, and olives.
7. Add pasta, sautéing until heated through.
8. To serve, drizzle pasta with remaining olive oil and enjoy.

NUTRITION: Calories: 207.4; Carbs: 31g; Protein: 5.1g; Fat: 7g

172. **Quinoa & Black Bean Stuffed Sweet Potatoes**

Servings: 8,

Cooking Time: 60 minutes

INGREDIENTS

- 4 sweet potatoes

- ½ onion, diced
- 1 garlic glove, crushed and diced
- ½ large bell pepper diced (about 2/3 cups)
- Handful of diced cilantro
- ½ cup cooked quinoa
- ½ cup black beans
- 1 tbsp olive oil
- 1 tbsp chili powder
- ½ tbsp cumin
- ½ tbsp paprika
- ½ tbsp oregano
- 2 tbsp lime juice
- 2 tbsp honey
- Sprinkle salt
- 1 cup shredded cheddar cheese
- Chopped spring onions, for garnish (optional)

DIRECTIONS

1. Preheat oven to 400oF.
2. Wash and scrub outside of potatoes. Poke with fork a few times and then place on parchment paper on cookie sheet. Bake for 40-45 minutes or until it is cooked.
3. While potatoes are baking, sauté onions, garlic, olive oil and spices in a pan on the stove until onions are translucent and soft.
4. In the last 10 minutes while the potatoes are cooking, in a large bowl combine the onion mixture with the beans, quinoa, honey, lime juice, cilantro and ½ cup cheese. Mix well.
5. When potatoes are cooked, remove from oven and let cool slightly. When cool to touch, cut in half (hot dog style) and scoop out most of the insides. Leave a thin ring of potato so that it will hold its shape. You can save the sweet potato guts for another recipe,

such as my veggie burgers (recipe posted below).
6. Fill with bean and quinoa mixture. Top with remaining cheddar cheese.
7. (If making this a freezer meal, stop here. Individually wrap potato skins in plastic wrap and place on flat surface to freeze. Once frozen, place all potatoes in large zip lock container or Tupperware.)
8. Return to oven for an additional 10 minutes or until cheese is melted.

NUTRITION: Calories: 243; Carbs: 37.6g; Protein: 8.5g; Fat: 7.3g

173. Quinoa and Three Beans Recipe

Servings: 8,

Cooking Time: 35 minutes

INGREDIENTS

- 1 cup grape tomatoes, sliced in half
- 1 cup quinoa
- 1 cup seedless cucumber, chopped
- 1 red bell pepper, seeds removed and chopped
- 1 tablespoon balsamic vinegar
- 1 yellow bell pepper, seeds removed and chopped
- 1/2-pound green beans, trimmed and snapped into 2-inch pieces
- 1/3 cup pitted kalamata olives, cut in half
- 1/4 cup chopped fresh basil
- 1/4 cup diced red onion
- 1/4 cup feta cheese crumbles
- 1/4 cup olive oil
- 1/4 teaspoon dried basil
- 1/4 teaspoon dried oregano

- 15 ounces garbanzo beans, drained and rinsed
- 15 ounces white beans, drained and rinsed
- 2 cups water
- 2 garlic cloves, smashed
- kosher salt and freshly ground black pepper to taste

DIRECTIONS

1. Bring water and quinoa to a boil in a medium saucepan. Cover, reduce heat to low, and cook until quinoa is tender, around 15 minutes.
2. Remove from heat and let stand for 5 minutes, covered.
3. Remove lid and fluff with a fork. Transfer to a large salad bowl.
4. Meanwhile. Bring a large pot of salted water to a boil and blanch the green beans for two minutes. Drain and place in a bowl of ice water. Drain well.
5. Add the fresh basil, olives, feta cheese, red onion, tomatoes, cucumbers, peppers, white beans, garbanzo beans, and green beans in bowl of quinoa.
6. In a small bowl, whisk together the pepper, salt, oregano, dried basil, balsamic, and olive oil. Pour dressing over the salad and gently toss salad until coated with dressing.
7. Season with additional salt and pepper if needed.
8. Serve and enjoy.

NUTRITION:Calories: 249; Carbs: 31.0g; Protein: 8.0g; Fat: 10.0g

174. <u>Quinoa Buffalo Bites</u>

Servings: 4,

Cooking Time: 15 minutes

INGREDIENTS

- 2 cups cooked quinoa
- 1 cup shredded mozzarella
- 1/2 cup buffalo sauce
- 1/4 cup +1 Tbsp flour
- 1 egg
- 1/4 cup chopped cilantro
- 1 small onion, diced

DIRECTIONS

1. Preheat oven to 350oF.
2. Mix all ingredients in large bowl.
3. Press mixture into greased mini muffin tins.
4. Bake for approximately 15 minutes or until bites are golden.
5. Enjoy on its own or with blue cheese or ranch dip.

NUTRITION:Calories: 212; Carbs: 30.6g; Protein: 15.9g; Fat: 3.0g

175. <u>Raisins, Nuts and Beef on Hashweh Rice</u>

Servings: 8,

Cooking Time: 50 minutes

INGREDIENTS

- ½ cup dark raisins, soaked in 2 cups water for an hour
- 1/3 cup slivered almonds, toasted and soaked in 2 cups water overnight

- 1/3 cup pine nuts, toasted and soaked in 2 cups water overnight
- ½ cup fresh parsley leaves, roughly chopped
- Pepper and salt to taste
- ¾ tsp ground cinnamon, divided
- ¾ tsp cloves, divided
- 1 tsp garlic powder
- 1 ¾ tsp allspice, divided
- 1 lb. lean ground beef or lean ground lamb
- 1 small red onion, finely chopped
- Olive oil
- 1 ½ cups medium grain rice

DIRECTIONS

1. For 15 to 20 minutes, soak rice in cold water. You will know that soaking is enough when you can snap a grain of rice easily between your thumb and index finger. Once soaking is done, drain rice well.
2. Meanwhile, drain pine nuts, almonds and raisins for at least a minute and transfer to one bowl. Set aside.
3. On a heavy cooking pot on medium high fire, heat 1 tbsp olive oil.
4. Once oil is hot, add red onions. Sauté for a minute before adding ground meat and sauté for another minute.
5. Season ground meat with pepper, salt, ½ tsp ground cinnamon, ½ tsp ground cloves, 1 tsp garlic powder, and 1 ¼ tsp allspice.
6. Sauté ground meat for 10 minutes or until browned and cooked fully. Drain fat.
7. In same pot with cooked ground meat, add rice on top of meat.
8. Season with a bit of pepper and salt. Add remaining cinnamon, ground cloves, and allspice. Do not mix.

9. Add 1 tbsp olive oil and 2 ½ cups of water. Bring to a boil and once boiling, lower fire to a simmer. Cook while covered until liquid is fully absorbed, around 20 to 25 minutes.
10. Turn of fire.
11. To serve, place a large serving platter that fully covers the mouth of the pot. Place platter upside down on mouth of pot, and invert pot. The inside of the pot should now rest on the platter with the rice on bottom of plate and ground meat on top of it.
12. Garnish the top of the meat with raisins, almonds, pine nuts, and parsley.
13. Serve and enjoy.

NUTRITION: Calories: 357; Carbs: 39.0g; Protein: 16.7g; Fat: 15.9g

176. Raw Tomato Sauce & Brie on Linguine

Servings: 4,

Cooking Time: 12 minutes

INGREDIENTS

- ¼ cup grated low-fat Parmesan cheese
- ½ cup loosely packed fresh basil leaves, torn
- 12 oz whole wheat linguine
- 2 cups loosely packed baby arugula
- 2 green onions, green parts only, sliced thinly
- 2 tbsp balsamic vinegar
- 2 tbsp extra virgin olive oil
- 3 large vine-ripened tomatoes
- 3 oz low-fat Brie cheese, cubed, rind removed and discarded

- 3 tbsp toasted pine nuts
- Pepper and salt to taste

DIRECTIONS

1. Toss together pepper, salt, vinegar, oil, onions, Parmesan, basil, arugula, Brie and tomatoes in a large bowl and set aside.
2. Cook linguine following package instructions. Reserve 1 cup of pasta cooking water after linguine is cooked. Drain and discard the rest of the pasta. Do not run under cold water, instead immediately add into bowl of salad. Let it stand for a minute without mixing.
3. Add ¼ cup of reserved pasta water into bowl to make a creamy sauce. Add more pasta water if desired. Toss to mix well.
4. Serve and enjoy.

NUTRITION: Calories: 274.7; Carbs: 30.9g; Protein: 14.6g; Fat: 10.3g

177. **Red Quinoa Peach Porridge**

Servings: 1,

Cooking Time: 30 minutes

INGREDIENTS

- ¼ cup old fashioned rolled oats
- ¼ cup red quinoa
- ½ cup milk
- 1 ½ cups water
- 2 peaches, peeled and sliced

DIRECTIONS

1. On a small saucepan, place the peaches and quinoa. Add water and cook for 30 minutes.
2. Add the oatmeal and milk last and cook until the oats become tender.
3. Stir occasionally to avoid the porridge from sticking on the bottom of the pan.

NUTRITION: Calories: 456.6; Carbs: 77.3g; Protein: 16.6g; Fat: 9g

178. **Red Wine Risotto**

Servings: 8,

Cooking Time: 25 minutes

INGREDIENTS

- Pepper to taste
- 1 cup finely shredded Parmigian-Reggiano cheese, divided
- 2 tsp tomato paste
- 1 ¾ cups dry red wine
- ¼ tsp salt
- 1 ½ cups Italian 'risotto' rice
- 2 cloves garlic, minced
- 1 medium onion, freshly chopped
- 2 tbsp extra-virgin olive oil
- 4 ½ cups reduced sodium beef broth

DIRECTIONS

1. On medium high fire, bring to a simmer broth in a medium fry pan. Lower fire so broth is steaming but not simmering.
2. On medium low heat, place a Dutch oven and heat oil.
3. Sauté onions for 5 minutes. Add garlic and cook for 2 minutes.

4. Add rice, mix well, and season with salt.
5. Into rice, add a generous splash of wine and ½ cup of broth.
6. Lower fire to a gentle simmer, cook until liquid is fully absorbed while stirring rice every once in a while.
7. Add another splash of wine and ½ cup of broth. Stirring once in a while.
8. Add tomato paste and stir to mix well.
9. Continue cooking and adding wine and broth until broth is used up.
10. Once done cooking, turn off fire and stir in pepper and ¾ cup cheese.
11. To serve, sprinkle with remaining cheese and enjoy.

NUTRITION:Calories: 231; Carbs: 33.9g; Protein: 7.9g; Fat: 5.7g

179. **Rice & Currant Salad Mediterranean Style**

Servings: 4,

Cooking Time: 50 minutes

INGREDIENTS

- 1 cup basmati rice
- salt
- 2 1/2 Tablespoons lemon juice
- 1 teaspoon grated orange zest
- 2 Tablespoons fresh orange juice
- 1/4 cup olive oil
- 1/2 teaspoon cinnamon
- Salt and pepper to taste
- 4 chopped green onions
- 1/2 cup dried currants
- 3/4 cup shelled pistachios or almonds
- 1/4 cup chopped fresh parsley

DIRECTIONS

1. Place a nonstick pot on medium high fire and add rice. Toast rice until opaque and starts to smell, around 10 minutes.
2. Add 4 quarts of boiling water to pot and 2 tsp salt. Boil until tender, around 8 minutes uncovered.
3. Drain the rice and spread out on a lined cookie sheet to cool completely.
4. In a large salad bowl, whisk well the oil, juices and spices. Add salt and pepper to taste.
5. Add half of the green onions, half of parsley, currants, and nuts.
6. Toss with the cooled rice and let stand for at least 20 minutes.
7. If needed adjust seasoning with pepper and salt.
8. Garnish with remaining parsley and green onions.

NUTRITION:Calories: 450; Carbs: 50.0g; Protein: 9.0g; Fat: 24.0g

180. **Ricotta and Spinach Ravioli**

Servings: 2,

Cooking Time: 15 minutes

INGREDIENTS

- 1 cup chicken stock
- 1 cup frozen spinach, thawed
- 1 batch pasta dough

INGREDIENTS Filling

- 3 tbsp heavy cream
- 1 cup ricotta
- 1 ¾ cups baby spinach

- 1 small onion, finely chopped
- 2 tbsp butter

DIRECTIONS

1. Create the filling: In a fry pan, sauté onion and butter around five minutes. Add the baby spinach leaves and continue simmering for another four minutes. Remove from fire, drain liquid and mince the onion and leaves. Then combine with 2 tbsp cream and the ricotta ensuring that it is well combined. Add pepper and salt to taste.
2. With your pasta dough, divide it into four balls. Roll out one ball to ¼ inch thick rectangular spread. Cut a 1 ½ inch by 3-inch rectangles. Place filling on the middle of the rectangles, around 1 tablespoonful and brush filling with cold water. Fold the rectangles in half, ensuring that no air is trapped within and seal using a cookie cutter. Use up all the filling.
3. Create Pasta Sauce: Until smooth, puree chicken stock and spinach. Pour into heated fry pan and for two minutes cook it. Add 1 tbsp cream and season with pepper and salt. Continue cooking for a minute and turn of fire.
4. Cook the raviolis by submerging in a boiling pot of water with salt. Cook until al dente then drain. Then quickly transfer the cooked ravioli into the fry pan of pasta sauce, toss to mix and serve.

NUTRITION: Calories: 443; Carbs: 12.3g; Protein: 18.8g; Fat: 36.8g

181. <u>Roasted Red Peppers and Shrimp Pasta</u>

Servings: 6,

Cooking Time: 10 minutes

INGREDIENTS

- 12 oz pasta, cooked and drained
- 1 cup finely shredded Parmesan Cheese
- ¼ cup snipped fresh basil
- ½ cup whipping cream
- ½ cup dry white wine
- 1 12oz jar roasted red sweet peppers, drained and chopped
- ¼ tsp crushed red pepper
- 6 cloves garlic, minced
- 1/3 cup finely chopped onion
- 2 tbsp olive oil
- ¼ cup butter
- 1 ½ lbs. fresh, peeled, deveined, rinsed and drained medium shrimps

DIRECTIONS

1. On medium high fire, heat butter in a big fry pan and add garlic and onions. Stir fry until onions are soft, around two minutes. Add crushed red pepper and shrimps, sauté for another two minutes before adding wine and roasted peppers.
2. Allow mixture to boil before lowering heat to low fire and for two minutes, let the mixture simmer uncovered. Stirring occasionally, add cream once shrimps are cooked and simmer for a minute.
3. Add basil and remove from fire. Toss in the pasta and mix gently. Transfer to serving plates and top with cheese.

NUTRITION: Calories: 418; Carbs: 26.9g; Protein: 37.1g; Fat: 18.8g

182. Seafood and Veggie Pasta

Servings: 4,

Cooking Time: 20 minutes

INGREDIENTS

- ¼ tsp pepper
- ¼ tsp salt
- 1 lb raw shelled shrimp
- 1 lemon, cut into wedges
- 1 tbsp butter
- 1 tbsp olive oil
- 2 5-oz cans chopped clams, drained (reserve 2 tbsp clam juice)
- 2 tbsp dry white wine
- 4 cloves garlic, minced
- 4 cups zucchini, spiraled (use a veggie spiralizer)
- 4 tbsp Parmesan Cheese
- Chopped fresh parsley to garnish

DIRECTIONS

1. Ready the zucchini and spiralize with a veggie spiralizer. Arrange 1 cup of zucchini noodle per bowl. Total of 4 bowls.
2. On medium fire, place a large nonstick saucepan and heat oil and butter.
3. For a minute, sauté garlic. Add shrimp and cook for 3 minutes until opaque or cooked.
4. Add white wine, reserved clam juice and clams. Bring to a simmer and continue simmering for 2 minutes or until half of liquid has evaporated. Stir constantly.

5. Season with pepper and salt. And if needed add more to taste.
6. Remove from fire and evenly distribute seafood sauce to 4 bowls.
7. Top with a tablespoonful of Parmesan cheese per bowl, serve and enjoy.

NUTRITION: Calories: 324.9; Carbs: 12g; Protein: 43.8g; Fat: 11.3g

183. Seafood Paella with Couscous

Servings: 4,

Cooking Time: 15 minutes

INGREDIENTS

- ½ cup whole wheat couscous
- 4 oz small shrimp, peeled and deveined
- 4 oz bay scallops, tough muscle removed
- ¼ cup vegetable broth
- 1 cup freshly diced tomatoes and juice
- Pinch of crumbled saffron threads
- ¼ tsp freshly ground pepper
- ¼ tsp salt
- ½ tsp fennel seed
- ½ tsp dried thyme
- 1 clove garlic, minced
- 1 medium onion, chopped
- 2 tsp extra virgin olive oil

DIRECTIONS

1. Put on medium fire a large saucepan and add oil. Stir in the onion and sauté for three minutes before adding: saffron, pepper, salt, fennel seed, thyme, and garlic. Continue to sauté for another minute.

2. Then add the broth and tomatoes and let boil. Once boiling, reduce the fire, cover and continue to cook for another 2 minutes.

3. Add the scallops and increase fire to medium and stir occasionally and cook for two minutes. Add the shrimp and wait for two minutes more before adding the couscous. Then remove from fire, cover and set aside for five minutes before carefully mixing.

NUTRITION: Calories: 117; Carbs: 11.7g; Protein: 11.5g; Fat: 3.1g

184. Shrimp Paella Made with Quinoa

Servings: 7,

Cooking Time: 40 minutes

INGREDIENTS

- 1 lb. large shrimp, peeled, deveined and thawed
- 1 tsp seafood seasoning
- 1 cup frozen green peas
- 1 red bell pepper, cored, seeded & membrane removed, sliced into ½" strips
- ½ cup sliced sun-dried tomatoes, packed in olive oil
- Salt to taste
- ½ tsp black pepper
- ½ tsp Spanish paprika
- ½ tsp saffron threads (optional turmeric)
- 1 bay leaf
- ¼ tsp crushed red pepper flakes
- 3 cups chicken broth, fat free, low sodium
- 1 ½ cups dry quinoa, rinse well

- 1 tbsp olive oil
- 2 cloves garlic, minced
- 1 yellow onion, diced

DIRECTIONS

1. Season shrimps with seafood seasoning and a pinch of salt. Toss to mix well and refrigerate until ready to use.

2. Prepare and wash quinoa. Set aside.

3. On medium low fire, place a large nonstick skillet and heat oil. Add onions and for 5 minutes sauté until soft and tender.

4. Add paprika, saffron (or turmeric), bay leaves, red pepper flakes, chicken broth and quinoa. Season with salt and pepper.

5. Cover skillet and bring to a boil. Once boiling, lower fire to a simmer and cook until all liquid is absorbed, around ten minutes.

6. Add shrimp, peas and sun-dried tomatoes. For 5 minutes, cover and cook.

7. Once done, turn off fire and for ten minutes allow paella to set while still covered.

8. To serve, remove bay leaf and enjoy with a squeeze of lemon if desired.

NUTRITION: Calories: 324.4; Protein: 22g; Carbs: 33g; Fat: 11.6g

185. Shrimp, Lemon and Basil Pasta

Servings: 4,

Cooking Time: 25 minutes

INGREDIENTS

- 2 cups baby spinach
- ½ tsp salt
- 2 tbsp fresh lemon juice
- 2 tbsp extra virgin olive oil
- 3 tbsp drained capers
- ¼ cup chopped fresh basil
- 1 lb. peeled and deveined large shrimp
- 8 oz uncooked spaghetti
- 3 quarts water

DIRECTIONS

1. In a pot, bring to boil 3 quarts water. Add the pasta and allow to boil for another eight mins before adding the shrimp and boiling for another three mins or until pasta is cooked.
2. Drain the pasta and transfer to a bowl. Add salt, lemon juice, olive oil, capers and basil while mixing well.
3. To serve, place baby spinach on plate around ½ cup and topped with ½ cup of pasta.

NUTRITION: Calories: 151; Carbs: 18.9g; Protein: 4.3g; Fat: 7.4g

186. <u>Simple Penne Anti-Pasto</u>

Servings: 4,

Cooking Time: 15 minutes

INGREDIENTS

- ¼ cup pine nuts, toasted
- ½ cup grated Parmigiano-Reggiano cheese, divided
- 8oz penne pasta, cooked and drained
- 1 6oz jar drained, sliced, marinated and quartered artichoke hearts
- 1 7 oz jar drained and chopped sun-dried tomato halves packed in oil
- 3 oz chopped prosciutto
- 1/3 cup pesto
- ½ cup pitted and chopped Kalamata olives
- 1 medium red bell pepper

DIRECTIONS

1. Slice bell pepper, discard membranes, seeds and stem. On a foiled lined baking sheet, place bell pepper halves, press down by hand and broil in oven for eight minutes. Remove from oven, put in a sealed bag for 5 minutes before peeling and chopping.
2. Place chopped bell pepper in a bowl and mix in artichokes, tomatoes, prosciutto, pesto and olives.
3. Toss in ¼ cup cheese and pasta. Transfer to a serving dish and garnish with ¼ cup cheese and pine nuts. Serve and enjoy!

NUTRITION: Calories: 606; Carbs: 70.3g; Protein: 27.2g; Fat: 27.6g

187. <u>Spaghetti in Lemon Avocado White Sauce</u>

Servings: 6,

Cooking Time: 30 minutes

INGREDIENTS

- Freshly ground black pepper
- Zest and juice of 1 lemon
- 1 avocado, pitted and peeled
- 1-pound spaghetti
- Salt
- 1 tbsp Olive oil
- 8 oz small shrimp, shelled and deveined

- ¼ cup dry white wine
- 1 large onion, finely sliced

DIRECTIONS

1. Let a big pot of water boil. Once boiling add the spaghetti or pasta and cook following manufacturer's instructions until al dente. Drain and set aside.
2. In a large fry pan, over medium fire sauté wine and onions for ten minutes or until onions are translucent and soft.
3. Add the shrimps into the fry pan and increase fire to high while constantly sautéing until shrimps are cooked around five minutes. Turn the fire off. Season with salt and add the oil right away. Then quickly toss in the cooked pasta, mix well.
4. In a blender, until smooth, puree the lemon juice and avocado. Pour into the fry pan of pasta, combine well. Garnish with pepper and lemon zest then serve.

NUTRITION: Calories: 206; Carbs: 26.3g; Protein: 10.2g; Fat: 8.0g

188. Spanish Rice Casserole with Cheesy Beef

Servings: 2,

Cooking Time: 32 minutes

INGREDIENTS

- 2 tablespoons chopped green bell pepper
- 1/4 teaspoon Worcestershire sauce
- 1/4 teaspoon ground cumin
- 1/4 cup shredded Cheddar cheese
- 1/4 cup finely chopped onion
- 1/4 cup chile sauce
- 1/3 cup uncooked long grain rice
- 1/2-pound lean ground beef
- 1/2 teaspoon salt
- 1/2 teaspoon brown sugar
- 1/2 pinch ground black pepper
- 1/2 cup water
- 1/2 (14.5 ounce) can canned tomatoes
- 1 tablespoon chopped fresh cilantro

DIRECTIONS

1. Place a nonstick saucepan on medium fire and brown beef for 10 minutes while crumbling beef. Discard fat.
2. Stir in pepper, Worcestershire sauce, cumin, brown sugar, salt, chile sauce, rice, water, tomatoes, green bell pepper, and onion. Mix well and cook for 10 minutes until blended and a bit tender.
3. Transfer to an ovenproof casserole and press down firmly. Sprinkle cheese on top and cook for 7 minutes at 400oF preheated oven. Broil for 3 minutes until top is lightly browned.
4. Serve and enjoy with chopped cilantro.

NUTRITION: Calories: 460; Carbohydrates: 35.8g; Protein: 37.8g; Fat: 17.9g

189. Squash and Eggplant Casserole

Servings: 2,

Cooking Time: 45 minutes

Vegetable INGREDIENTS

- ½ cup dry white wine

- 1 eggplant, halved and cut to 1-inch slices
- 1 large onion, cut into wedges
- 1 red bell pepper, seeded and cut to julienned strips
- 1 small butternut squash, cut into 1-inch slices
- 1 tbsp olive oil
- 12 baby corn
- 2 cups low sodium vegetable broth
- Salt and pepper to taste
- Polenta Ingredients
- ¼ cup parmesan cheese, grated
- 1 cup instant polenta
- 2 tbsp fresh oregano, chopped
- Topping Ingredients
- 1 garlic clove, chopped
- 2 tbsp slivered almonds
- 5 tbsp parsley, chopped
- Grated zest of 1 lemon

DIRECTIONS

1. Preheat the oven to 350 degrees Fahrenheit.
2. In a casserole, heat the oil and add the onion wedges and baby corn. Sauté over medium high heat for five minutes. Stir occasionally to prevent the onions and baby corn from sticking at the bottom of the pan.
3. Add the butternut squash to the casserole and toss the vegetables. Add the eggplants and the red pepper.
4. Cover the vegetables and cook over low to medium heat.
5. Cook for about ten minutes before adding the wine. Let the wine sizzle before stirring in the broth. Bring to a boil and cook in the oven for 30 minutes.
6. While the casserole is cooking inside the oven, make the topping by spreading the slivered almonds on a baking tray and toasting under the grill until they are lightly browned.
7. Place the toasted almonds in a small bowl and mix the remaining ingredients for the toppings.
8. Prepare the polenta. In a large saucepan, bring 3 cups of water to boil over high heat.
9. Add the polenta and continue whisking until it absorbs all the water.
10. Reduce the heat to medium until the polenta is thick. Add the parmesan cheese and oregano.
11. Serve the polenta on plates and add the casserole on top. Sprinkle the toppings on top.

NUTRITION:Calories: 579.3; Carbs: 79.2g; Protein: 22.2g; Fat: 19.3g

190. Stuffed Tomatoes with Green Chili

Servings: 6,

Cooking Time: 55 minutes

INGREDIENTS

- 4 oz Colby-Jack shredded cheese
- ¼ cup water
- 1 cup uncooked quinoa
- 6 large ripe tomatoes
- ¼ tsp freshly ground black pepper
- ¾ tsp ground cumin
- 1 tsp salt, divided
- 1 tbsp fresh lime juice
- 1 tbsp olive oil
- 1 tbsp chopped fresh oregano
- 1 cup chopped onion
- 2 cups fresh corn kernels
- 2 poblano chilies

DIRECTIONS

1. Preheat broiler to high.
2. Slice lengthwise the chilies and press on a baking sheet lined with foil. Broil for 8 minutes. Remove from oven and let cool for 10 minutes. Peel the chilies and chop coarsely and place in medium sized bowl.
3. Place onion and corn in baking sheet and broil for ten minutes. Stir two times while broiling. Remove from oven and mix in with chopped chilies.
4. Add black pepper, cumin, ¼ tsp salt, lime juice, oil and oregano. Mix well.
5. Cut off the tops of tomatoes and set aside. Leave the tomato shell intact as you scoop out the tomato pulp.
6. Drain tomato pulp as you press down with a spoon. Reserve 1 ¼ cups of tomato pulp liquid and discard the rest. Invert the tomato shells on a wire rack for 30 mins and then wipe the insides dry with a paper towel.
7. Season with ½ tsp salt the tomato pulp.
8. On a sieve over a bowl, place quinoa. Add water until it covers quinoa. Rub quinoa grains for 30 seconds together with hands; rinse and drain. Repeat this procedure two times and drain well at the end.
9. In medium saucepan bring to a boil remaining salt, ¼ cup water, quinoa and tomato liquid.
10. Once boiling, reduce heat and simmer for 15 minutes or until liquid is fully absorbed. Remove from heat and fluff quinoa with fork. Transfer and mix well the quinoa with the corn mixture.
11. Spoon ¾ cup of the quinoa-corn mixture into the tomato shells, top with cheese and cover with the tomato top. Bake in a preheated 350oF oven for

15 minutes and then broil high for another 1.5 minutes.

NUTRITION: Calories: 276; Carbs: 46.3g; Protein: 13.4g; Fat: 4.1g

191. Tasty Lasagna Rolls

Servings: 6,

Cooking Time: 20 minutes

INGREDIENTS

- ¼ tsp crushed red pepper
- ¼ tsp salt
- ½ cup shredded mozzarella cheese
- ½ cups parmesan cheese, shredded
- 1 14-oz package tofu, cubed
- 1 25-oz can of low-sodium marinara sauce
- 1 tbsp extra virgin olive oil
- 12 whole wheat lasagna noodles
- 2 tbsp Kalamata olives, chopped
- 3 cloves minced garlic
- 3 cups spinach, chopped

DIRECTIONS

1. Put enough water on a large pot and cook the lasagna noodles according to package instructions. Drain, rinse and set aside until ready to use.
2. In a large skillet, sauté garlic over medium heat for 20 seconds. Add the tofu and spinach and cook until the spinach wilts. Transfer this mixture in a bowl and add parmesan olives, salt, red pepper and 2/3 cup of the marinara sauce.
3. In a pan, spread a cup of marinara sauce on the bottom. To make the rolls, place noodle on a surface and spread ¼ cup of the tofu filling. Roll up

and place it on the pan with the marinara sauce. Do this procedure until all lasagna noodles are rolled.

4. Place the pan over high heat and bring to a simmer. Reduce the heat to medium and let it cook for three more minutes. Sprinkle mozzarella cheese and let the cheese melt for two minutes. Serve hot.

NUTRITION: Calories: 304; Carbs: 39.2g; Protein: 23g; Fat: 19.2g

192. <u>Tasty Mushroom Bolognese</u>

Servings: 6,

Cooking Time: 65 minutes

INGREDIENTS

- ¼ cup chopped fresh parsley
  - oz Parmigiano-Reggiano cheese, grated
- 1 tbsp kosher salt
- 10-oz whole wheat spaghetti, cooked and drained
- ¼ cup milk
- 1 14-oz can whole peeled tomatoes
- ½ cup white wine
- 2 tbsp tomato paste
- 1 tbsp minced garlic
- 8 cups finely chopped cremini mushrooms
- ½ lb. ground pork
- ½ tsp freshly ground black pepper, divided
- ¾ tsp kosher salt, divided
- 2 ½ cups chopped onion
- 1 tbsp olive oil
- 1 cup boiling water
- ½-oz dried porcini mushrooms

DIRECTIONS

1. Let porcini stand in a boiling bowl of water for twenty minutes, drain (reserve liquid), rinse and chop. Set aside.
2. On medium high fire, place a Dutch oven with olive oil and cook for ten minutes cook pork, ¼ tsp pepper, ¼ tsp salt and onions. Constantly mix to break ground pork pieces.
3. Stir in ¼ tsp pepper, ¼ tsp salt, garlic and cremini mushrooms. Continue cooking until liquid has evaporated, around fifteen minutes.
4. Stirring constantly, add porcini and sauté for a minute.
5. Stir in wine, porcini liquid, tomatoes and tomato paste. Let it simmer for forty minutes. Stir occasionally. Pour milk and cook for another two minutes before removing from fire.
6. Stir in pasta and transfer to a serving dish. Garnish with parsley and cheese before serving.

NUTRITION: Calories: 358; Carbs: 32.8g; Protein: 21.1g; Fat: 15.4g

193. <u>Tortellini Salad with Broccoli</u>

Servings: 12,

Cooking Time: 20 minutes

INGREDIENTS

- 1 red onion, chopped finely
- 1 cup sunflower seeds
- 1 cup raisins
- 3 heads fresh broccoli, cut into florets
- 2 tsp cider vinegar
- ½ cup white sugar

- ½ cup mayonnaise
- 20-oz fresh cheese filled tortellini

DIRECTIONS

1. In a large pot of boiling water, cook tortellini according to manufacturer's instructions. Drain and rinse with cold water and set aside.
2. Whisk vinegar, sugar and mayonnaise to create your salad dressing.
3. Mix together in a large bowl red onion, sunflower seeds, raisins, tortellini and broccoli. Pour dressing and toss to coat.
4. Serve and enjoy.

NUTRITION: Calories: 272; Carbs: 38.7g; Protein: 5.0g; Fat: 8.1g

194. Turkey and Quinoa Stuffed Peppers

Servings: 6,

Cooking Time: 55 minutes

INGREDIENTS

- 3 large red bell peppers
- 2 tsp chopped fresh rosemary
- 2 tbsp chopped fresh parsley
- 3 tbsp chopped pecans, toasted
- ¼ cup extra virgin olive oil
- ½ cup chicken stock
- ½ lb. fully cooked smoked turkey sausage, diced
- ½ tsp salt
- 2 cups water
- 1 cup uncooked quinoa

DIRECTIONS

1. On high fire, place a large saucepan and add salt, water and quinoa. Bring to a boil.
2. Once boiling, reduce fire to a simmer, cover and cook until all water is absorbed around 15 minutes.
3. Uncover quinoa, turn off fire and let it stand for another 5 minutes.
4. Add rosemary, parsley, pecans, olive oil, chicken stock and turkey sausage into pan of quinoa. Mix well.
5. Slice peppers lengthwise in half and discard membranes and seeds. In another boiling pot of water, add peppers, boil for 5 minutes, drain and discard water.
6. Grease a 13 x 9 baking dish and preheat oven to 350oF.
7. Place boiled bell pepper onto prepared baking dish, evenly fill with the quinoa mixture and pop into oven.

Bake for 15 minutes.

NUTRITION: Calories: 255.6; Carbs: 21.6g; Protein: 14.4g; Fat: 12.4g

195. Veggie Pasta with Shrimp, Basil and Lemon

Servings: 4,

Cooking Time: 5 minutes

INGREDIENTS

- 2 cups baby spinach
- ½ tsp salt
- 2 tbsp fresh lemon juice
- 2 tbsp extra virgin olive oil
- 3 tbsp drained capers
- ¼ cup chopped fresh basil

- 1 lb. peeled and deveined large shrimp
- 4 cups zucchini, spirals

DIRECTIONS

1. divide into 4 serving plates, top with ¼ cup of spinach, serve and enjoy.

NUTRITION: Calories: 51; Carbs: 4.4g; Protein: 1.8g; Fat: 3.4g

196. Veggies and Sun-Dried Tomato Alfredo

Servings: 4,

Cooking Time: 30 minutes

INGREDIENTS

- 2 tsp finely shredded lemon peel
- ½ cup finely shredded Parmesan cheese
- 1 ¼ cups milk
- 2 tbsp all-purpose flour
- 8 fresh mushrooms, sliced
- 1 ½ cups fresh broccoli florets
- 4 oz fresh trimmed and quartered Brussels sprouts
- 4 oz trimmed fresh asparagus spears
- 1 tbsp olive oil
- 4 tbsp butter
- ½ cup chopped dried tomatoes
- 8 oz dried fettuccine

DIRECTIONS

1. In a boiling pot of water, add fettuccine and cook following manufacturer's instructions. Two minutes before the pasta is cooked, add the dried tomatoes. Drain pasta and tomatoes and return to pot to keep warm. Set aside.

2. On medium high fire, in a big fry pan with 1 tbsp butter, fry mushrooms, broccoli, Brussels sprouts and asparagus. Cook for eight minutes while covered, transfer to a plate and put aside.

3. Using same fry pan, add remaining butter and flour. Stirring vigorously, cook for a minute or until thickened. Add Parmesan cheese, milk and mix until cheese is melted around five minutes.

4. Toss in the pasta and mix. Transfer to serving dish. Garnish with Parmesan cheese and lemon peel before serving.

NUTRITION: Calories: 439; Carbs: 52.0g; Protein: 16.3g; Fat: 19.5g

197. Yangchow Chinese Style Fried Rice

Servings: 4,
Cooking Time: 20 minutes

INGREDIENTS

- 4 cups cold cooked rice
- 1/2 cup peas
- 1 medium yellow onion, diced
- 5 tbsp olive oil
- 4 oz frozen medium shrimp, thawed, shelled, deveined and chopped finely
- 6 oz roast pork
- 3 large eggs
- Salt and freshly ground black pepper
- 1/2 tsp cornstarch

DIRECTIONS

1. Combine the salt and ground black pepper and 1/2 tsp cornstarch, coat the shrimp with it. Chop the roasted pork. Beat the eggs and set aside.

2. Stir-fry the shrimp in a wok on high fire with 1 tbsp heated oil until pink, around 3 minutes. Set the shrimp aside and stir fry the roasted pork briefly. Remove both from the pan.

3. In the same pan, stir-fry the onion until soft, Stir the peas and cook until bright green. Remove both from pan.

4. Add 2 tbsp oil in the same pan, add the cooked rice. Stir and separate the individual grains. Add the beaten eggs, toss the rice. Add the roasted pork, shrimp, vegetables and onion. Toss everything together. Season with salt and pepper to taste.

NUTRITION: Calories: 556; Carbs: 60.2g; Protein: 20.2g; Fat: 25.2g

SEAFOOD & FISH RECIPES

198. Mediterranean Fish Fillets

Preparation Time: 10 minutes

Cooking Time: 3 minutes

Servings: 4

INGREDIENTS

- 4 cod fillets
- 1 lb grape tomatoes, halved
- 1 cup olives, pitted and sliced
- 2 tbsp capers
- 1 tsp dried thyme
- 2 tbsp olive oil
- 1 tsp garlic, minced
- Pepper
- Salt

DIRECTIONS

1. Pour 1 cup water into the instant pot then place steamer rack in the pot.
2. Spray heat-safe baking dish with cooking spray.
3. Add half grape tomatoes into the dish and season with pepper and salt.
4. Arrange fish fillets on top of cherry tomatoes. Drizzle with oil and season with garlic, thyme, capers, pepper, and salt.
5. Spread olives and remaining grape tomatoes on top of fish fillets.
6. Place dish on top of steamer rack in the pot.
7. Seal pot with a lid and select manual and cook on high for 3 minutes.
8. Once done, release pressure using quick release. Remove lid.
9. Serve and enjoy.

NUTRITION: Calories 212 Fat 11.9 g Carbohydrates 7.1 g Sugar 3 g Protein 21.4 g Cholesterol 55 mg

199. Flavors Cioppino

Preparation Time: 10 minutes

Cooking Time: 5 minutes

Servings: 6

INGREDIENTS

- 1 lb codfish, cut into chunks
- 1 1/2 lbs shrimp
- 28 oz can tomatoes, diced
- 1 cup dry white wine
- 1 bay leaf
- 1 tsp cayenne
- 1 tsp oregano
- 1 shallot, chopped
- 1 tsp garlic, minced
- 1 tbsp olive oil
- 1/2 tsp salt

DIRECTIONS

1. Add oil into the inner pot of instant pot and set the pot on sauté mode.
2. Add shallot and garlic and sauté for 2 minutes.
3. Add wine, bay leaf, cayenne, oregano, and salt and cook for 3 minutes.
4. Add remaining ingredients and stir well.
5. Seal pot with a lid and select manual and cook on low for 0 minutes.

6. Once done, release pressure using quick release. Remove lid.
7. Serve and enjoy.

NUTRITION: Calories 281 Fat 5 g Carbohydrates 10.5 g Sugar 4.9 g Protein 40.7 g Cholesterol 266 mg

200. Delicious Shrimp Alfredo

Preparation Time: 10 minutes

Cooking Time: 3 minutes

Servings: 4

INGREDIENTS

- 12 shrimp, remove shells
- 1 tbsp garlic, minced
- 1/4 cup parmesan cheese
- 2 cups whole wheat rotini noodles
- 1 cup fish broth
- 15 oz alfredo sauce
- 1 onion, chopped
- Salt

DIRECTIONS

1. Add all ingredients except parmesan cheese into the instant pot and stir well.
2. Seal pot with lid and cook on high for 3 minutes.
3. Once done, release pressure using quick release. Remove lid.
4. Stir in cheese and serve.

NUTRITION: Calories 669 Fat 23.1 g Carbohydrates 76 g Sugar 2.4 g Protein 37.8 g Cholesterol 190 mg

201. Tomato Olive Fish Fillets

Preparation Time: 10 minutes

Cooking Time: 8 minutes

Servings: 4

INGREDIENTS

- 2 lbs halibut fish fillets
- 2 oregano sprigs
- 2 rosemary sprigs
- 2 tbsp fresh lime juice
- 1 cup olives, pitted
- 28 oz can tomatoes, diced
- 1 tbsp garlic, minced
- 1 onion, chopped
- 2 tbsp olive oil

DIRECTIONS

1. Add oil into the inner pot of instant pot and set the pot on sauté mode.
2. Add onion and sauté for 3 minutes.
3. Add garlic and sauté for a minute.
4. Add lime juice, olives, herb sprigs, and tomatoes and stir well.
5. Seal pot with lid and cook on high for 3 minutes.
6. Once done, release pressure using quick release. Remove lid.
7. Add fish fillets and seal pot again with lid and cook on high for 2 minutes.
8. Once done, release pressure using quick release. Remove lid.
9. Serve and enjoy.

NUTRITION: Calories 333 Fat 19.1 g Carbohydrates 31.8 g Sugar 8.4 g Protein 13.4 g Cholesterol 5 mg

202. Shrimp Scampi

Preparation Time: 10 minutes

Cooking Time: 8 minutes

Servings: 6

INGREDIENTS

- 1 lb whole wheat penne pasta
- 1 lb frozen shrimp
- 2 tbsp garlic, minced
- 1/4 tsp cayenne
- 1/2 tbsp Italian seasoning
- 1/4 cup olive oil
- 3 1/2 cups fish stock
- Pepper
- Salt

DIRECTIONS

1. Add all ingredients into the inner pot of instant pot and stir well.
2. Seal pot with lid and cook on high for 6 minutes.
3. Once done, release pressure using quick release. Remove lid.
4. Stir well and serve.

NUTRITION: Calories 435 Fat 12.6 g Carbohydrates 54.9 g Sugar 0.1 g Protein 30.6 g Cholesterol 116 mg

203. Easy Salmon Stew

Preparation Time: 10 minutes

Cooking Time: 8 minutes

Servings: 6

INGREDIENTS

- 2 lbs salmon fillet, cubed
- 1 onion, chopped
- 2 cups fish broth
- 1 tbsp olive oil
- Pepper
- salt

DIRECTIONS

1. Add oil into the inner pot of instant pot and set the pot on sauté mode.
2. Add onion and sauté for 2 minutes.
3. Add remaining ingredients and stir well.
4. Seal pot with lid and cook on high for 6 minutes.
5. Once done, release pressure using quick release. Remove lid.
6. Stir and serve.

NUTRITION: Calories 243 Fat 12.6 g Carbohydrates 0.8 g Sugar 0.3 g Protein 31 g Cholesterol 78 mg

204. Italian Tuna Pasta

Preparation Time: 10 minutes

Cooking Time: 5 minutes

Servings: 6

INGREDIENTS

- 15 oz whole wheat pasta
- 2 tbsp capers
- 3 oz tuna
- 2 cups can tomatoes, crushed
- 2 anchovies
- 1 tsp garlic, minced
- 1 tbsp olive oil
- Salt

DIRECTIONS

1. Add oil into the inner pot of instant pot and set the pot on sauté mode.
2. Add anchovies and garlic and sauté for 1 minute.
3. Add remaining ingredients and stir well. Pour enough water into the pot to cover the pasta.
4. Seal pot with a lid and select manual and cook on low for 4 minutes.
5. Once done, release pressure using quick release. Remove lid.
6. Stir and serve.

NUTRITION: Calories 339 Fat 6 g Carbohydrates 56.5 g Sugar 5.2 g Protein 15.2 g Cholesterol 10 mg

205. Garlicky Clams

Preparation Time: 10 minutes

Cooking Time: 5 minutes

Servings: 4

INGREDIENTS

- 3 lbs clams, clean
- 4 garlic cloves
- 1/4 cup olive oil
- 1/2 cup fresh lemon juice
- 1 cup white wine
- Pepper
- Salt

DIRECTIONS

1. Add oil into the inner pot of instant pot and set the pot on sauté mode.
2. Add garlic and sauté for 1 minute.
3. Add wine and cook for 2 minutes.

4. Add remaining ingredients and stir well.
5. Seal pot with lid and cook on high for 2 minutes.
6. Once done, allow to release pressure naturally. Remove lid.
7. Serve and enjoy.

NUTRITION: Calories 332 Fat 13.5 g Carbohydrates 40.5 g Sugar 12.4 g Protein 2.5 g Cholesterol 0 mg

206. Delicious Fish Tacos

Preparation Time: 10 minutes

Cooking Time: 8 minutes

Servings: 8

INGREDIENTS

- 4 tilapia fillets
- 1/4 cup fresh cilantro, chopped
- 1/4 cup fresh lime juice
- 2 tbsp paprika
- 1 tbsp olive oil
- Pepper
- Salt

DIRECTIONS

1. Pour 2 cups of water into the instant pot then place steamer rack in the pot.
2. Place fish fillets on parchment paper.
3. Season fish fillets with paprika, pepper, and salt and drizzle with oil and lime juice.
4. Fold parchment paper around the fish fillets and place them on a steamer rack in the pot.
5. Seal pot with lid and cook on high for 8 minutes.

6. Once done, release pressure using quick release. Remove lid.
7. Remove fish packet from pot and open it.
8. Shred the fish with a fork and serve.

NUTRITION: Calories 67 Fat 2.5 g Carbohydrates 1.1 g Sugar 0.2 g Protein 10.8 g Cholesterol 28 mg

207. Pesto Fish Fillet

Preparation Time: 10 minutes

Cooking Time: 8 minutes

Servings: 4

INGREDIENTS

- 4 halibut fillets
- 1/2 cup water
- 1 tbsp lemon zest, grated
- 1 tbsp capers
- 1/2 cup basil, chopped
- 1 tbsp garlic, chopped
- 1 avocado, peeled and chopped
- Pepper
- Salt

DIRECTIONS

1. Add lemon zest, capers, basil, garlic, avocado, pepper, and salt into the blender blend until smooth.
2. Place fish fillets on aluminum foil and spread a blended mixture on fish fillets.
3. Fold foil around the fish fillets.
4. Pour water into the instant pot and place trivet in the pot.
5. Place foil fish packet on the trivet.
6. Seal pot with lid and cook on high for 8 minutes.

7. Once done, allow to release pressure naturally. Remove lid.
8. Serve and enjoy.

NUTRITION: Calories 426 Fat 16.6 g Carbohydrates 5.5 g Sugar 0.4 g Protein 61.8 g Cholesterol 93 mg

208. Tuna Risotto

Preparation Time: 10 minutes

Cooking Time: 23 minutes

Servings: 6

INGREDIENTS

- 1 cup of rice
- 1/3 cup parmesan cheese, grated
- 1 1/2 cups fish broth
- 1 lemon juice
- 1 tbsp garlic, minced
- 1 onion, chopped
- 2 tbsp olive oil
- 2 cups can tuna, cut into chunks
- Pepper
- Salt

DIRECTIONS

1. Add oil into the inner pot of instant pot and set the pot on sauté mode.
2. Add garlic, onion, and tuna and cook for 3 minutes.
3. Add remaining ingredients except for parmesan cheese and stir well.
4. Seal pot with lid and cook on high for 20 minutes.
5. Once done, release pressure using quick release. Remove lid.
6. Stir in parmesan cheese and serve.

NUTRITION: Calories 228 Fat 7 g Carbohydrates 27.7 g Sugar 1.2 g Protein 12.6 g Cholesterol 21 mg

209. <u>Salsa Fish Fillets</u>

Preparation Time: 10 minutes

Cooking Time: 2 minutes

Servings: 4

INGREDIENTS

- 1 lb tilapia fillets
- 1/2 cup salsa
- 1 cup of water
- Pepper
- Salt

DIRECTIONS

1. Place fish fillets on aluminum foil and top with salsa and season with pepper and salt.
2. Fold foil around the fish fillets.
3. Pour water into the instant pot and place trivet in the pot.
4. Place foil fish packet on the trivet.
5. Seal pot with lid and cook on high for 2 minutes.
6. Once done, release pressure using quick release. Remove lid.
7. Serve and enjoy.

NUTRITION: Calories 342 Fat 10.5 g Carbohydrates 41.5 g Sugar 1.9 g Protein 18.9 g Cholesterol 31 mg

210. **Coconut Clam Chowder**

Preparation Time: 10 minutes

Cooking Time: 7 minutes

Servings: 6

INGREDIENTS

- 6 oz clams, chopped
- 1 cup heavy cream
- 1/4 onion, sliced
- 1 cup celery, chopped
- 1 lb cauliflower, chopped
- 1 cup fish broth
- 1 bay leaf
- 2 cups of coconut milk
- Salt

DIRECTIONS

1. Add all ingredients except clams and heavy cream and stir well.
2. Seal pot with lid and cook on high for 5 minutes.
3. Once done, release pressure using quick release. Remove lid.
4. Add heavy cream and clams and stir well and cook on sauté mode for 2 minutes.
5. Stir well and serve.

NUTRITION: Calories 301 Fat 27.2 g Carbohydrates 13.6 g Sugar 6 g Protein 4.9 g Cholesterol 33 mg

211. **Feta Tomato Sea Bass**

Preparation Time: 10 minutes

Cooking Time: 8 minutes

Servings: 4

INGREDIENTS

- 4 sea bass fillets
- 1 1/2 cups water
- 1 tbsp olive oil

- 1 tsp garlic, minced
- 1 tsp basil, chopped
- 1 tsp parsley, chopped
- 1/2 cup feta cheese, crumbled
- 1 cup can tomatoes, diced
- Pepper
- Salt

DIRECTIONS

1. Season fish fillets with pepper and salt.
2. Pour 2 cups of water into the instant pot then place steamer rack in the pot.
3. Place fish fillets on steamer rack in the pot.
4. Seal pot with lid and cook on high for 5 minutes.
5. Once done, release pressure using quick release. Remove lid.
6. Remove fish fillets from the pot and clean the pot.
7. Add oil into the inner pot of instant pot and set the pot on sauté mode.
8. Add garlic and sauté for 1 minute.
9. Add tomatoes, parsley, and basil and stir well and cook for 1 minute.
10. Add fish fillets and top with crumbled cheese and cook for a minute.
11. Serve and enjoy.

NUTRITION: Calories 219 Fat 10.1 g Carbohydrates 4 g Sugar 2.8 g Protein 27.1 g Cholesterol 70 mg

212. Stewed Mussels & Scallops

Preparation Time: 10 minutes

Cooking Time: 11 minutes

Servings: 4

INGREDIENTS

- 2 cups mussels
- 1 cup scallops
- 2 cups fish stock
- 2 bell peppers, diced
- 2 cups cauliflower rice
- 1 onion, chopped
- 1 tbsp olive oil
- Pepper
- Salt

DIRECTIONS

1. Add oil into the inner pot of instant pot and set the pot on sauté mode.
2. Add onion and peppers and sauté for 3 minutes.
3. Add scallops and cook for 2 minutes.
4. Add remaining ingredients and stir well.
5. Seal pot with lid and cook on high for 6 minutes.
6. Once done, allow to release pressure naturally. Remove lid.
7. Stir and serve.

NUTRITION: Calories 191 Fat 7.4 g Carbohydrates 13.7 g Sugar 6.2 g Protein 18 g

Cholesterol 29 mg

213. Healthy Halibut Soup

Preparation Time: 10 minutes

Cooking Time: 13 minutes

Servings: 4

INGREDIENTS

- 1 lb halibut, skinless, boneless, & cut into chunks
- 2 tbsp ginger, minced
- 2 celery stalks, chopped
- 1 carrot, sliced
- 1 onion, chopped
- 1 cup of water
- 2 cups fish stock
- 1 tbsp olive oil
- Pepper
- Salt

DIRECTIONS

1. Add oil into the inner pot of instant pot and set the pot on sauté mode.
2. Add onion and sauté for 3-4 minutes.
3. Add water, celery, carrot, ginger, and stock and stir well.
4. Seal pot with lid and cook on high for 5 minutes.
5. Once done, release pressure using quick release. Remove lid.
6. Add fish and stir well. Seal pot again and cook on high for 4 minutes.
7. Once done, release pressure using quick release. Remove lid.
8. Stir and serve.

NUTRITION: Calories 4586 Fat 99.6 g Carbohydrates 6.3 g Sugar 2.1 g Protein 861 g Cholesterol 1319 mg

214. **Creamy Fish Stew**

Preparation Time: 10 minutes

Cooking Time: 8 minutes

Servings: 6

INGREDIENTS

- 1 lb white fish fillets, cut into chunks
- 2 tbsp olive oil
- 1 cup kale, chopped
- 1 cup cauliflower, chopped
- 1 cup broccoli, chopped
- 3 cups fish broth
- 1 cup heavy cream
- 2 celery stalks, diced
- 1 carrot, sliced
- 1 onion, diced
- Pepper
- Salt

DIRECTIONS

1. Add oil into the inner pot of instant pot and set the pot on sauté mode.
2. Add onion and sauté for 3 minutes.
3. Add remaining ingredients except for heavy cream and stir well.
4. Seal pot with lid and cook on high for 5 minutes.
5. Once done, allow to release pressure naturally. Remove lid.
6. Stir in heavy cream and serve.

NUTRITION: Calories 296 Fat 19.3 g Carbohydrates 7.5 g Sugar 2.6 g Protein 22.8 g Cholesterol 103 mg

215. **Nutritious Broccoli Salmon**

Preparation Time: 10 minutes

Cooking Time: 4 minutes

Servings: 4

INGREDIENTS

- 4 salmon fillets
- 10 oz broccoli florets

- 1 1/2 cups water
- 1 tbsp olive oil
- Pepper
- Salt

DIRECTIONS

1. Pour water into the instant pot then place steamer basket in the pot.
2. Place salmon in the steamer basket and season with pepper and salt and drizzle with oil.
3. Add broccoli on top of salmon in the steamer basket.
4. Seal pot with lid and cook on high for 4 minutes.
5. Once done, release pressure using quick release. Remove lid.
6. Serve and enjoy.

NUTRITION: Calories 290 Fat 14.7 g Carbohydrates 4.7 g Sugar 1.2 g Protein 36.5 g Cholesterol 78 mg

216. Shrimp Zoodles

Preparation Time: 10 minutes

Cooking Time: 5 minutes

Servings: 4

INGREDIENTS

- 2 zucchini, spiralized
- 1 lb shrimp, peeled and deveined
- 1/2 tsp paprika
- 1 tbsp basil, chopped
- 1/2 lemon juice
- 1 tsp garlic, minced
- 2 tbsp olive oil
- 1 cup vegetable stock
- Pepper
- Salt

DIRECTIONS

1. Add oil into the inner pot of instant pot and set the pot on sauté mode.
2. Add garlic and sauté for a minute.
3. Add shrimp and lemon juice and stir well and cook for 1 minute.
4. Add remaining ingredients and stir well.
5. Seal pot with lid and cook on high for 3 minutes.
6. Once done, release pressure using quick release. Remove lid.
7. Serve and enjoy.

NUTRITION: Calories 215 Fat 9.2 g Carbohydrates 5.8 g Sugar 2 g Protein 27.3 g Cholesterol 239 mg

217. Healthy Carrot & Shrimp

Preparation Time: 10 minutes

Cooking Time: 6 minutes

Servings: 4

INGREDIENTS

- 1 lb shrimp, peeled and deveined
- 1 tbsp chives, chopped
- 1 onion, chopped
- 1 tbsp olive oil
- 1 cup fish stock
- 1 cup carrots, sliced
- Pepper
- Salt

DIRECTIONS

1. Add oil into the inner pot of instant pot and set the pot on sauté mode.
2. Add onion and sauté for 2 minutes.
3. Add shrimp and stir well.

4. Add remaining ingredients and stir well.
5. Seal pot with lid and cook on high for 4 minutes.
6. Once done, release pressure using quick release. Remove lid.
7. Serve and enjoy.

NUTRITION: Calories 197 Fat 5.9 g Carbohydrates 7 g Sugar 2.5 g Protein 27.7 g Cholesterol 239 mg

218. **Salmon with Potatoes**

Preparation Time: 10 minutes

Cooking Time: 15 minutes

Servings: 4

INGREDIENTS

- 1 1/2 lbs Salmon fillets, boneless and cubed
- 2 tbsp olive oil
- 1 cup fish stock
- 2 tbsp parsley, chopped
- 1 tsp garlic, minced
- 1 lb baby potatoes, halved
- Pepper
- Salt

DIRECTIONS

1. Add oil into the inner pot of instant pot and set the pot on sauté mode.
2. Add garlic and sauté for 2 minutes.
3. Add remaining ingredients and stir well.
4. Seal pot with lid and cook on high for 13 minutes.
5. Once done, release pressure using quick release. Remove lid.
6. Serve and enjoy.

NUTRITION: Calories 362 Fat 18.1 g Carbohydrates 14.5 g Sugar 0 g Protein 37.3 g Cholesterol 76 mg

219. **Honey Garlic Shrimp**

Preparation Time: 10 minutes

Cooking Time: 5 minutes

Servings: 4

INGREDIENTS

- 1 lb shrimp, peeled and deveined
- 1/4 cup honey
- 1 tbsp garlic, minced
- 1 tbsp ginger, minced
- 1 tbsp olive oil
- 1/4 cup fish stock
- Pepper
- Salt

DIRECTIONS

1. Add shrimp into the large bowl. Add remaining ingredients over shrimp and toss well.
2. Transfer shrimp into the instant pot and stir well.
3. Seal pot with lid and cook on high for 5 minutes.
4. Once done, release pressure using quick release. Remove lid.
5. Serve and enjoy.

NUTRITION: Calories 240 Fat 5.6 g Carbohydrates 20.9 g Sugar 17.5 g Protein 26.5 g Cholesterol 239 mg

220. **Simple Lemon Clams**

Preparation Time: 10 minutes

Cooking Time: 10 minutes

Servings: 4

INGREDIENTS

- 1 lb clams, clean
- 1 tbsp fresh lemon juice
- 1 lemon zest, grated
- 1 onion, chopped
- 1/2 cup fish stock
- Pepper
- Salt

DIRECTIONS

1. Add all ingredients into the inner pot of instant pot and stir well.
2. Seal pot with lid and cook on high for 10 minutes.
3. Once done, release pressure using quick release. Remove lid.
4. Serve and enjoy.

NUTRITION: Calories 76 Fat 0.6 g Carbohydrates 16.4 g Sugar 5.4 g Protein 1.8 g Cholesterol 0 mg

221. Crab Stew

Preparation Time: 10 minutes

Cooking Time: 13 minutes

Servings: 2

INGREDIENTS

- 1/2 lb lump crab meat
- 2 tbsp heavy cream
- 1 tbsp olive oil
- 2 cups fish stock
- 1/2 lb shrimp, shelled and chopped
- 1 celery stalk, chopped

- 1/2 tsp garlic, chopped
- 1/4 onion, chopped
- Pepper
- Salt

DIRECTIONS

1. Add oil into the inner pot of instant pot and set the pot on sauté mode.
2. Add onion and sauté for 3 minutes.
3. Add garlic and sauté for 30 seconds.
4. Add remaining ingredients except for heavy cream and stir well.
5. Seal pot with lid and cook on high for 10 minutes.
6. Once done, release pressure using quick release. Remove lid.
7. Stir in heavy cream and serve.

NUTRITION: Calories 376 Fat 25.5 g Carbohydrates 5.8 g Sugar 0.7 g Protein 48.1 g Cholesterol 326 mg

222. Honey Balsamic Salmon

Preparation Time: 10 minutes

Cooking Time: 3 minutes

Servings: 2

INGREDIENTS

- 2 salmon fillets
- 1/4 tsp red pepper flakes
- 2 tbsp honey
- 2 tbsp balsamic vinegar
- 1 cup of water
- Pepper
- Salt

DIRECTIONS

1. Pour water into the instant pot and place trivet in the pot.
2. In a small bowl, mix together honey, red pepper flakes, and vinegar.
3. Brush fish fillets with honey mixture and place on top of the trivet.
4. Seal pot with lid and cook on high for 3 minutes.
5. Once done, release pressure using quick release. Remove lid.
6. Serve and enjoy.

NUTRITION: Calories 303 Fat 11 g Carbohydrates 17.6 g Sugar 17.3 g Protein 34.6 g Cholesterol 78 mg

223. Spicy Tomato Crab Mix

Preparation Time: 10 minutes

Cooking Time: 12 minutes

Servings: 4

INGREDIENTS

- 1 lb crab meat
- 1 tsp paprika
- 1 cup grape tomatoes, cut into half
- 2 tbsp green onion, chopped
- 1 tbsp olive oil
- Pepper
- Salt

DIRECTIONS

1. Add oil into the inner pot of instant pot and set the pot on sauté mode.
2. Add paprika and onion and sauté for 2 minutes.
3. Add the rest of the ingredients and stir well.

4. Seal pot with lid and cook on high for 10 minutes.
5. Once done, release pressure using quick release. Remove lid.
6. Serve and enjoy.

NUTRITION: Calories 142 Fat 5.7 g Carbohydrates 4.3 g Sugar 1.3 g Protein 14.7 g Cholesterol 61 mg

224. Dijon Fish Fillets

Preparation Time: 10 minutes

Cooking Time: 3 minutes

Servings: 2

INGREDIENTS

- 2 white fish fillets
- 1 tbsp Dijon mustard
- 1 cup of water
- Pepper
- Salt

DIRECTIONS

1. Pour water into the instant pot and place trivet in the pot.
2. Brush fish fillets with mustard and season with pepper and salt and place on top of the trivet.
3. Seal pot with lid and cook on high for 3 minutes.
4. Once done, release pressure using quick release. Remove lid.
5. Serve and enjoy.

NUTRITION: Calories 270 Fat 11.9 g Carbohydrates 0.5 g Sugar 0.1 g Protein 38 g Cholesterol 119 mg

225. **Lemoney Prawns**

Preparation Time: 10 minutes

Cooking Time: 3 minutes

Servings: 2

INGREDIENTS

- 1/2 lb prawns
- 1/2 cup fish stock
- 1 tbsp fresh lemon juice
- 1 tbsp lemon zest, grated
- 1 tbsp olive oil
- 1 tbsp garlic, minced
- Pepper
- Salt

DIRECTIONS

1. Add all ingredients into the inner pot of instant pot and stir well.
2. Seal pot with lid and cook on high for 3 minutes.
3. Once done, release pressure using quick release. Remove lid.
4. Drain prawns and serve.

NUTRITION: Calories 215 Fat 9.5 g Carbohydrates 3.9 g Sugar 0.4 g Protein 27.6 g Cholesterol 239 mg

226. **Lemon Cod Peas**

Preparation Time: 10 minutes

Cooking Time: 10 minutes

Servings: 4

INGREDIENTS

- 1 lb cod fillets, skinless, boneless and cut into chunks
- 1 cup fish stock
- 1 tbsp fresh parsley, chopped
- 1/2 tbsp lemon juice
- 1 green chili, chopped
- 3/4 cup fresh peas
- 2 tbsp onion, chopped
- Pepper
- Salt

DIRECTIONS

1. Add all ingredients into the inner pot of instant pot and stir well.
2. Seal pot with lid and cook on high for 10 minutes.
3. Once done, release pressure using quick release. Remove lid.
4. Stir and serve.

NUTRITION: Calories 128 Fat 1.6 g Carbohydrates 5 g Sugar 2.1 g Protein 23.2 g Cholesterol 41 mg

227. **Quick & Easy Shrimp**

Preparation Time: 10 minutes

Cooking Time: 1 minute

Servings: 6

DIRECTIONS

- 1 3/4 lbs shrimp, frozen and deveined
- 1/2 cup fish stock
- 1/2 cup apple cider vinegar
- Pepper
- Salt

DIRECTIONS

1. Add all ingredients into the inner pot of instant pot and stir well.
2. Seal pot with lid and cook on high for 1 minute.
3. Once done, release pressure using quick release. Remove lid.
4. Stir and serve.

NUTRITION: Calories 165 Fat 2.4 g Carbohydrates 2.2 g Sugar 0.1 g Protein 30.6 g Cholesterol 279 mg

228. Creamy Curry Salmon

Preparation time: 10 minutes

Cooking time: 20 minutes

Servings: 2

INGREDIENTS

- 2 salmon fillets, boneless and cubed
- 1 tablespoon olive oil
- 1 tablespoon basil, chopped
- Sea salt and black pepper to the taste
- 1 cup Greek yogurt
- 2 teaspoons curry powder
- 1 garlic clove, minced
- ½ teaspoon mint, chopped

DIRECTIONS

1. Heat up a pan with the oil over medium-high heat, add the salmon and cook for 3 minutes.
2. Add the rest of the ingredients, toss, cook for 15 minutes more, divide between plates and serve.

NUTRITION: Calories 284, fat 14.1, fiber 8.5, carbs 26.7, protein 31.4

229. Mahi Mahi and Pomegranate Sauce

Preparation time: 10 minutes

Cooking time: 10 minutes

Servings: 4

INGREDIENTS

- 1 and ½ cups chicken stock
- 1 tablespoon olive oil
- 4 mahi mahi fillets, boneless
- 4 tablespoons tahini paste
- Juice of 1 lime
- Seeds from 1 pomegranate
- 1 tablespoon parsley, chopped

DIRECTIONS

1. Heat up a pan with the oil over medium-high heat, add the fish and cook for 3 minutes on each side.
2. Add the rest of the ingredients, flip the fish again, cook for 4 minutes more, divide everything between plates and serve.

NUTRITION: Calories 224, fat 11.1, fiber 5.5, carbs 16.7, protein 11.4

230. Smoked Salmon and Veggies Mix

Preparation time: 10 minutes

Cooking time: 20 minutes

Servings: 4

INGREDIENTS

- 3 red onions, cut into wedges

- ¾ cup green olives, pitted and halved
- 3 red bell peppers, roughly chopped
- ½ teaspoon smoked paprika
- Salt and black pepper to the taste
- 3 tablespoons olive oil
- 4 salmon fillets, skinless and boneless
- 2 tablespoons chives, chopped

DIRECTIONS

1. In a roasting pan, combine the salmon with the onions and the rest of the ingredients, introduce in the oven and bake at 390 degrees F for 20 minutes.
2. Divide the mix between plates and serve.

NUTRITION: Calories 301, fat 5.9, fiber 11.9, carbs 26.4, protein 22.4

231. Salmon and Mango Mix

Preparation time: 10 minutes

Cooking time: 25 minutes

Servings: 2

INGREDIENTS

- 2 salmon fillets, skinless and boneless
- Salt and pepper to the taste
- 2 tablespoons olive oil
- 2 garlic cloves, minced
- 2 mangos, peeled and cubed
- 1 red chili, chopped
- 1 small piece ginger, grated
- Juice of 1 lime
- 1 tablespoon cilantro, chopped

DIRECTIONS

1. In a roasting pan, combine the salmon with the oil, garlic and the rest of the

ingredients except the cilantro, toss, introduce in the oven at 350 degrees F and bake for 25 minutes.
2. Divide everything between plates and serve with the cilantro sprinkled on top.

NUTRITION: Calories 251, fat 15.9, fiber 5.9, carbs 26.4, protein 12.4

232. Salmon and Creamy Endives

Preparation time: 10 minutes

Cooking time: 15 minutes

Servings: 4

INGREDIENTS

- 4 salmon fillets, boneless
- 2 endives, shredded
- Juice of 1 lime
- Salt and black pepper to the taste
- ¼ cup chicken stock
- 1 cup Greek yogurt
- ¼ cup green olives pitted and chopped
- ¼ cup fresh chives, chopped
- 3 tablespoons olive oil

DIRECTIONS

1. Heat up a pan with half of the oil over medium heat, add the endives and the rest of the ingredients except the chives and the salmon, toss, cook for 6 minutes and divide between plates.
2. Heat up another pan with the rest of the oil, add the salmon, season with salt and pepper, cook for 4 minutes on each side, add next to the creamy

endives mix, sprinkle the chives on top and serve.

NUTRITION: Calories 266, fat 13.9, fiber 11.1, carbs 23.8, protein 17.5

233. <u>Trout and Tzatziki Sauce</u>

Preparation time: 10 minutes

Cooking time: 10 minutes

Servings: 4

INGREDIENTS

- Juice of ½ lime
- Salt and black pepper to the taste
- 1 and ½ teaspoon coriander, ground
- 1 teaspoon garlic, minced
- 4 trout fillets, boneless
- 1 teaspoon sweet paprika
- 2 tablespoons avocado oil
- For the sauce:
- 1 cucumber, chopped
- 4 garlic cloves, minced
- 1 tablespoon olive oil
- 1 teaspoon white vinegar
- 1 and ½ cups Greek yogurt
- A pinch of salt and white pepper

DIRECTIONS

1. Heat up a pan with the avocado oil over medium-high heat, add the fish, salt, pepper, lime juice, 1 teaspoon garlic and the paprika, rub the fish gently and cook for 4 minutes on each side.
2. In a bowl, combine the cucumber with 4 garlic cloves and the rest of the ingredients for the sauce and whisk well.

3. Divide the fish between plates, drizzle the sauce all over and serve with a side salad.

NUTRITION: Calories 393, fat 18.5, fiber 6.5, carbs 18.3, protein 39.6

234. <u>Parsley Trout and Capers</u>

Preparation time: 10 minutes

Cooking time: 10 minutes

Servings: 4

INGREDIENTS

- 4 trout fillets, boneless
- 3 ounces tomato sauce
- A handful parsley, chopped
- 2 tablespoons olive oil
- Salt and black pepper to the taste

DIRECTIONS

1. Heat up a pan with the oil over medium-high heat, add the fish, salt and pepper and cook for 3 minutes on each side.
2. Add the rest of the ingredients, cook everything for 4 minutes more.
3. Divide everything between plates and serve.

NUTRITION: Calories 308, fat 17, fiber 1, carbs 3, protein 16

235. <u>Baked Trout and Fennel</u>

Preparation time: 10 minutes

Cooking time: 22 minutes

Servings: 4

INGREDIENTS

- 1 fennel bulb, sliced
- 2 tablespoons olive oil
- 1 yellow onion, sliced
- 3 teaspoons Italian seasoning
- 4 rainbow trout fillets, boneless
- ¼ cup panko breadcrumbs
- ½ cup kalamata olives, pitted and halved
- Juice of 1 lemon

DIRECTIONS

1. Spread the fennel the onion and the rest of the ingredients except the trout and the breadcrumbs on a baking sheet lined with parchment paper, toss them and cook at 400 degrees F for 10 minutes.
2. Add the fish dredged in breadcrumbs and seasoned with salt and pepper and cook it at 400 degrees F for 6 minutes on each side.
3. Divide the mix between plates and serve.

NUTRITION: Calories 306, fat 8.9, fiber 11.1, carbs 23.8, protein 14.5

236. Lemon Rainbow Trout

Preparation time: 10 minutes

Cooking time: 15 minutes

Servings: 2

INGREDIENTS

- 2 rainbow trout
- Juice of 1 lemon
- 3 tablespoons olive oil
- 4 garlic cloves, minced
- A pinch of salt and black pepper

DIRECTIONS

1. Line a baking sheet with parchment paper, add the fish and the rest of the ingredients and rub.
2. Bake at 400 degrees F for 15 minutes, divide between plates and serve with a side salad.

NUTRITION: Calories 521, fat 29, fiber 5, carbs 14, protein 52

237. Trout and Peppers Mix

Preparation time: 10 minutes

Cooking time: 20 minutes

Servings: 4

INGREDIENTS

- 4 trout fillets, boneless
- 2 tablespoons kalamata olives, pitted and chopped
- 1 tablespoon capers, drained
- 2 tablespoons olive oil
- A pinch of salt and black pepper
- 1 and ½ teaspoons chili powder
- 1 yellow bell pepper, chopped
- 1 red bell pepper, chopped
- 1 green bell pepper, chopped

DIRECTIONS

1. Heat up a pan with the oil over medium-high heat, add the trout, salt and pepper and cook for 10 minutes.
2. Flip the fish, add the peppers and the rest of the ingredients, cook for 10 minutes more, divide the whole mix between plates and serve.

NUTRITION: Calories 572, fat 17.4, fiber 6, carbs 71, protein 33.7

238. <u>Cod and Cabbage</u>

Preparation time: 10 minutes

Cooking time: 15 minutes

Servings: 4

INGREDIENTS

- 3 cups green cabbage, shredded
- 1 sweet onion, sliced
- A pinch of salt and black pepper
- ½ cup feta cheese, crumbled
- 4 teaspoons olive oil
- 4 cod fillets, boneless
- ¼ cup green olives, pitted and chopped

DIRECTIONS

1. Grease a roasting pan with the oil, add the fish, the cabbage and the rest of the ingredients, introduce in the pan and cook at 450 degrees F for 15 minutes.
2. Divide the mix between plates and serve.

NUTRITION: Calories 270, fat 10, fiber 3, carbs 12, protein 31

239. <u>Mediterranean Mussels</u>

Preparation time: 10 minutes

Cooking time: 10 minutes

Servings: 4

INGREDIENTS

- 1 white onion, sliced
- 3 tablespoons olive oil
- 2 teaspoons fennel seeds
- 4 garlic cloves, minced
- 1 teaspoon red pepper, crushed
- A pinch of salt and black pepper
- 1 cup chicken stock
- 1 tablespoon lemon juice
- 2 and ½ pounds mussels, scrubbed
- ½ cup parsley, chopped
- ½ cup tomatoes, cubed

DIRECTIONS

1. Heat up a pan with the oil over medium-high heat, add the onion and the garlic and sauté for 2 minutes.
2. Add the rest of the ingredients except the mussels, stir and cook for 3 minutes more.
3. Add the mussels, cook everything for 6 minutes more, divide everything into bowls and serve.

NUTRITION: Calories 276, fat 9.8, fiber 4.8, carbs 6.5, protein 20.5

240. <u>Mussels Bowls</u>

Preparation time: 10 minutes

Cooking time: 10 minutes

Servings: 4

INGREDIENTS

- 2 pounds mussels, scrubbed
- 1 tablespoon garlic, minced
- 1 tablespoon basil, chopped
- 1 yellow onion, chopped
- 6 tomatoes, cubed

- 1 cup heavy cream
- 2 tablespoons olive oil
- 1 tablespoon parsley, chopped

DIRECTIONS

1. Heat up a pan with the oil over medium-high heat, add the garlic and the onion and sauté for 2 minutes.
2. Add the mussels and the rest of the ingredients, toss, cook for 7 minutes more, divide into bowls and serve.

NUTRITION: Calories 266, fat 11.8, fiber 5.8, carbs 16.5, protein 10.5

241. Calamari and Dill Sauce

Preparation time: 10 minutes

Cooking time: 15 minutes

Servings: 4

INGREDIENTS

- 1 and ½ pound calamari, sliced into rings
- 10 garlic cloves, minced
- 2 tablespoons olive oil
- Juice of 1 and ½ lime
- 2 tablespoons balsamic vinegar
- 3 tablespoons dill, chopped
- A pinch of salt and black pepper

DIRECTIONS

1. Heat up a pan with the oil over medium-high heat, add the garlic, lime juice and the other ingredients except the calamari and cook for 5 minutes.
2. Add the calamari rings, cook everything for 10 minutes more, divide between plates and serve.

NUTRITION: Calories 282, fat 18.6, fiber 4, carbs 9.2, protein 18.5

242. Chili Calamari and Veggie Mix

Preparation time: 10 minutes

Cooking time: 40 minutes

Servings: 4

INGREDIENTS

- 1 pound calamari rings
- 2 red chili peppers, chopped
- 2 tablespoons olive oil
- 3 garlic cloves, minced
- 14 ounces canned tomatoes, chopped
- 2 tablespoons tomato paste
- 1 tablespoon thyme, chopped
- Salt and black pepper to the taste
- 2 tablespoons capers, drained
- 12 black olives, pitted and halved

DIRECTIONS

1. Heat up a pan with the oil over medium-high heat, add the garlic and the chili peppers and sauté for 2 minutes.
2. Add the rest of the ingredients except the olives and capers, stir, bring to a simmer and cook for 22 minutes.
3. Add the olives and capers, cook everything for 15 minutes more, divide everything into bowls and serve.

NUTRITION: Calories 274, fat 11.6, fiber 2.8, carbs 13.5, protein 15.4

243. Cheesy Crab and Lime Spread

Preparation time: 10 minutes

Cooking time: 25 minutes

Servings: 8

INGREDIENTS

1 pound crab meat, flaked

4 ounces cream cheese, soft

1 tablespoon chives, chopped

1 teaspoon lime juice

1 teaspoon lime zest, grated

DIRECTIONS

1. 350 degrees F, bake for 25 minutes, divide into bowls and serve.

NUTRITION: Calories 284, fat 14.6, fiber 5.8, carbs 16.5, protein 15.4

244. Horseradish Cheesy Salmon Mix

Preparation time: 1 hour

Cooking time: 0 minutes

Servings: 8

INGREDIENTS

- 2 ounces feta cheese, crumbled
- 4 ounces cream cheese, soft
- 3 tablespoons already prepared horseradish
- 1 pound smoked salmon, skinless, boneless and flaked
- 2 teaspoons lime zest, grated
- 1 red onion, chopped
- 3 tablespoons chives, chopped

DIRECTIONS

2. In your food processor, mix cream cheese with horseradish, goat cheese and lime zest and blend very well.
3. In a bowl, combine the salmon with the rest of the ingredients, toss and serve cold.

NUTRITION: Calories 281, fat 17.9, fiber 1, carbs 4.2, protein 25.3

245. Greek Trout Spread

Preparation time: 5 minutes

Cooking time: 0 minutes

Servings: 8

INGREDIENTS

- 4 ounces smoked trout, skinless, boneless and flaked
- 1 tablespoon lemon juice
- 1 cup Greek yogurt
- tablespoon dill, chopped
- Salt and black pepper to the taste
- A drizzle of olive oil

DIRECTIONS

1. In a bowl, combine the trout with the lemon juice and the rest of the ingredients and whisk really well.
2. Divide the spread into bowls and serve.

NUTRITION: Calories 258, fat 4,5, fiber 2, carbs 5.5, protein 7.6

246. Scallions and Salmon Tartar

Preparation time: 5 minutes

Cooking time: 0 minutes

Servings: 4

INGREDIENTS

- 4 tablespoons scallions, chopped
- 2 teaspoons lemon juice
- 1 tablespoon chives, minced
- 1 tablespoon olive oil
- 1 pound salmon, skinless, boneless and minced
- Salt and black pepper to the taste
- 1 tablespoon parsley, chopped

DIRECTIONS

In a bowl, combine the scallions with the salmon and the rest of the ingredients, stir well, divide into small moulds between plates and serve.

NUTRITION: Calories 224, fat 14.5, fiber 5.2, carbs 12.7, protein 5.3

247. Salmon and Green Beans

Preparation time: 10 minutes

Cooking time: 15 minutes

Servings: 4

INGREDIENTS

- 3 tablespoons balsamic vinegar
- 2 tablespoons olive oil
- 1 garlic clove, minced
- ½ teaspoons red pepper flakes, crushed
- ½ teaspoon lime zest, grated
- 1 and ½ pounds green beans, chopped
- Salt and black pepper to the taste
- 1 red onion, sliced
- 4 salmon fillets, boneless

DIRECTIONS

1. Heat up a pan with half of the oil, add the vinegar, onion, garlic and the other ingredients except the salmon, toss, cook for 6 minutes and divide between plates.
2. Heat up the same pan with the rest of the oil over medium-high heat, add the salmon, salt and pepper, cook for 4 minutes on each side, add next to the green beans and serve.

NUTRITION: Calories 224, fat 15.5, fiber 8.2, carbs 22.7, protein 16.3

248. Cayenne Cod and Tomatoes

Preparation time: 10 minutes

Cooking time: 25 minutes

Servings: 4

INGREDIENTS

- 1 teaspoon lime juice
- Salt and black pepper to the taste
- 1 teaspoon sweet paprika
- 1 teaspoon cayenne pepper
- 2 tablespoons olive oil
- 1 yellow onion, chopped
- 2 garlic cloves, minced
- 4 cod fillets, boneless

- A pinch of cloves, ground
- ½ cup chicken stock
- ½ pound cherry tomatoes, cubed

DIRECTIONS

1. Heat up a pan with the oil over medium-high heat add the cod, salt, pepper and the cayenne, cook for 4 minutes on each side and divide between plates.
2. Heat up the same pan over medium-high heat, add the onion and garlic and sauté for 5 minutes.
3. Add the rest of the ingredients, stir, bring to a simmer and cook for 10 minutes more.
4. Divide the mix next to the fish and serve.

NUTRITION: Calories 232, fat 16.5, fiber 11.1, carbs 24.8, protein 16.5

249. **Salmon and Watermelon Gazpacho**

Preparation time: 4 hours

Cooking time: 0 minutes

Servings: 4

INGREDIENTS

- ¼ cup basil, chopped
- 1 pound tomatoes, cubed
- 1 pound watermelon, cubed
- ¼ cup red wine vinegar
- 1/3 cup avocado oil
- 2 garlic cloves, minced
- 1 cup smoked salmon, skinless, boneless and cubed
- A pinch of salt and black pepper

DIRECTIONS

1. In your blender, combine the basil with the watermelon and the rest of the ingredients except the salmon, pulse well and divide into bowls.
2. Top each serving with the salmon and serve cold.

NUTRITION: Calories 252, fat 16.5, fiber 9.1, carbs 24.8, protein 15.5

250. **Shrimp and Calamari Mix**

Preparation time: 10 minutes

Cooking time: 12 minutes

Servings: 4

INGREDIENTS

- 1 pound shrimp, peeled and deveined
- Salt and black pepper to the taste
- 3 garlic cloves, minced
- 1 tablespoon avocado oil
- ½ pound calamari rings
- ½ teaspoon basil, dried
- 1 teaspoon rosemary, dried
- 1 red onion, chopped
- 1 cup chicken stock
- Juice of 1 lemon
- 1 tablespoon parsley, chopped

DIRECTIONS

1. Heat up a pan with the oil over medium-high heat, add the onion and the garlic and sauté for 4 minutes.
2. Add the shrimp, the calamari and the rest of the ingredients except the parsley, stir, bring to a simmer and cook for 8 minutes.

3. Add the parsley, divide everything into bowls and serve.

NUTRITION: Calories 288, fat 12.8, fiber 10.2, carbs 22.2, protein 6.8

251. Shrimp and Dill Mix

Preparation time: 10 minutes

Cooking time: 10 minutes

Servings: 4

- **INGREDIENTS**
- 1 pound shrimp, cooked, peeled and deveined
- ½ cup raisins
- 1 cup spring onion, chopped
- 2 tablespoons olive oil
- 2 tablespoons capers, chopped
- 2 tablespoons dill, chopped
- Salt and black pepper to the taste

DIRECTIONS

1. Heat up a pan with the oil over medium-high heat, add the onions and raisins and sauté for 2-3 minutes.
2. Add the shrimp and the rest of the ingredients, toss, cook for 6 minutes more, divide between plates and serve with a side salad.

NUTRITION: Calories 218, fat 12.8, fiber 6.2, carbs 22.2, protein 4.8

252. Minty Sardines Salad

Preparation time: 10 minutes

Cooking time: 0 minutes

Servings: 4

INGREDIENTS

- 4 ounces canned sardines in olive oil, skinless, boneless and flaked
- 2 teaspoons avocado oil
- 2 tablespoons mint, chopped
- A pinch of salt and black pepper
- 1 avocado, peeled, pitted and cubed
- 1 cucumber, cubed
- 2 tomatoes, cubed
- 2 spring onions, chopped

DIRECTIONS

In a bowl, combine the sardines with the oil and the rest of the ingredients, toss, divide into small cups and keep in the fridge for 10 minutes before serving.

NUTRITION: Calories 261, fat 7.6, fiber 2.2, carbs 22.8, protein 12.5

VEGETABLES

253. Potato Salad

Preparation Time: 10 minutes

Cooking Time: 10 minutes

Servings: 8

INGREDIENTS

- 5 cups potato, cubed
- 1/4 cup fresh parsley, chopped
- 1/4 tsp red pepper flakes
- 1 tbsp olive oil
- 1/3 cup mayonnaise
- 1/2 tbsp oregano
- 2 tbsp capers
- 3/4 cup feta cheese, crumbled
- 1 cup olives, halved
- 3 cups of water
- 3/4 cup onion, chopped
- Pepper
- Salt

DIRECTIONS

1. Add potatoes, onion, and salt into the instant pot.
2. Seal pot with lid and cook on high for 3 minutes.
3. Once done, release pressure using quick release. Remove lid.
4. Remove potatoes from pot and place in a large mixing bowl.
5. Add remaining ingredients and stir everything well.
6. Serve and enjoy.

NUTRITION: Calories 152 Fat 9.9 g Carbohydrates 13.6 g Sugar 2.1 g Protein 3.5 g Cholesterol 15 mg

254. Greek Green Beans

Preparation Time: 10 minutes

Cooking Time: 15 minutes

Servings: 4

INGREDIENTS

- 1 lb green beans, remove stems
- 2 potatoes, quartered
- 1 1/2 onion, sliced
- 1 tsp dried oregano
- 1/4 cup dill, chopped
- 1/4 cup fresh parsley, chopped
- 1 zucchini, quartered
- 1/2 cup olive oil
- 1 cup of water
- k14.5 oz can tomatoes, diced
- Pepper
- Salt

DIRECTIONS

1. Add all ingredients into the inner pot of instant pot and stir everything well.
2. Seal pot with lid and cook on high for 15 minutes.
3. Once done, release pressure using quick release. Remove lid.
4. Stir well and serve.

NUTRITION: Calories 381 Fat 25.8 g Carbohydrates 37.7 g Sugar 9 g Protein 6.6 g Cholesterol 0 mg

255. **Healthy Vegetable Medley**

Preparation Time: 10 minutes

Cooking Time: 17 minutes

Servings: 6

INGREDIENTS

- 3 cups broccoli florets
- 1 sweet potato, chopped
- 1 tsp garlic, minced
- 14 oz coconut milk
- 28 oz can tomatoes, chopped
- 14 oz can chickpeas, drained and rinsed
- 1 onion, chopped
- 1 tbsp olive oil
- 1 tsp Italian seasoning
- Pepper
- Salt

DIRECTIONS

1. Add oil into the inner pot of instant pot and set the pot on sauté mode.
2. Add garlic and onion and sauté until onion is softened.
3. Add remaining ingredients and stir everything well.
4. Seal pot with lid and cook on high for 12 minutes.
5. Once done, allow to release pressure naturally for 10 minutes then release remaining using quick release. Remove lid.
6. Stir well and serve.

NUTRITION: Calories 322 Fat 19.3 g Carbohydrates 34.3 g Sugar 9.6 g Protein 7.9 g Cholesterol 1 mg

256. **Spicy Zucchini**

Preparation Time: 10 minutes

Cooking Time: 5 minutes

Servings: 4

INGREDIENTS

- 4 zucchini, cut into 1/2-inch pieces
- 1 cup of water
- 1/2 tsp Italian seasoning
- 1/2 tsp red pepper flakes
- 1 tsp garlic, minced
- 1 tbsp olive oil
- 1/2 cup can tomato, crushed
- Salt

DIRECTIONS

1. Add water and zucchini into the instant pot.
2. Seal pot with lid and cook on high for 2 minutes.
3. Once done, release pressure using quick release. Remove lid.
4. Drain zucchini well and clean the instant pot.
5. Add oil into the inner pot of instant pot and set the pot on sauté mode.
6. Add garlic and sauté for 30 seconds.
7. Add remaining ingredients and stir well and cook for 2-3 minutes.
8. Serve and enjoy.

NUTRITION: Calories 69 Fat 4.1 g Carbohydrates 7.9 g Sugar 3.5 g Protein 2.7 g Cholesterol 0 mg

257. <u>Healthy Garlic Eggplant</u>

Preparation Time: 10 minutes

Cooking Time: 10 minutes

Servings: 4

INGREDIENTS

- 1 eggplant, cut into 1-inch pieces
- 1/2 cup water
- 1/4 cup can tomato, crushed
- 1/2 tsp Italian seasoning
- 1 tsp paprika
- 1/2 tsp chili powder
- 1 tsp garlic powder
- 2 tbsp olive oil
- Salt

DIRECTIONS

1. Add water and eggplant into the instant pot.
2. Seal pot with lid and cook on high for 5 minutes.
3. Once done, release pressure using quick release. Remove lid.
4. Drain eggplant well and clean the instant pot.
5. Add oil into the inner pot of instant pot and set the pot on sauté mode.
6. Add eggplant along with remaining ingredients and stir well and cook for 5 minutes.
7. Serve and enjoy.

NUTRITION: Calories 97 Fat 7.5 g Carbohydrates 8.2 g Sugar 3.7 g Protein 1.5 g Cholesterol 0 mg

258. <u>Carrot Potato Medley</u>

Preparation Time: 10 minutes

Cooking Time: 15 minutes

Servings: 6

INGREDIENTS

- 4 lbs baby potatoes, clean and cut in half
- 1 1/2 lbs carrots, cut into chunks
- 1 tsp Italian seasoning
- 1 1/2 cups vegetable broth
- 1 tbsp garlic, chopped
- 1 onion, chopped
- 2 tbsp olive oil
- Pepper
- Salt

DIRECTIONS

1. Add oil into the inner pot of instant pot and set the pot on sauté mode.
2. Add onion and sauté for 5 minutes.
3. Add carrots and cook for 5 minutes.
4. Add remaining ingredients and stir well.
5. Seal pot with lid and cook on high for 5 minutes.
6. Once done, allow to release pressure naturally for 10 minutes then release remaining using quick release. Remove lid.
7. Stir and serve.

NUTRITION: Calories 283 Fat 5.6 g Carbohydrates 51.3 g Sugar 6.6 g Protein 10.2 g Cholesterol 1 mg

259. <u>Lemon Herb Potatoes</u>

Preparation Time: 10 minutes

Cooking Time: 11 minutes

Servings: 6

INGREDIENTS

- 1 1/2 lbs baby potatoes, rinsed and pat dry
- 1/2 fresh lemon juice
- 1 tsp dried oregano
- 1/2 tsp garlic, minced
- 1 tbsp olive oil
- 1 cup vegetable broth
- 1/2 tsp sea salt

DIRECTIONS

1. Add broth and potatoes into the instant pot.
2. Seal pot with lid and cook on high for 8 minutes.
3. Once done, release pressure using quick release. Remove lid.
4. Drain potatoes well and clean the instant pot.
5. Add oil into the inner pot of instant pot and set the pot on sauté mode.
6. Add potatoes, garlic, oregano, lemon juice, and salt and cook for 3 minutes.
7. Serve and enjoy.

NUTRITION: Calories 94 Fat 2.7 g Carbohydrates 14.6 g Sugar 0.2 g Protein 3.8 g Cholesterol 0 mg

260. Flavors Basil Lemon Ratatouille

Preparation Time: 10 minutes

Cooking Time: 10 minutes

Servings: 8

INGREDIENTS

- 1 small eggplant, cut into cubes
- 1 cup fresh basil

- 2 cups grape tomatoes
- 1 onion, chopped
- 2 summer squash, sliced
- 2 zucchini, sliced
- 2 tbsp vinegar
- 2 tbsp tomato paste
- 1 tbsp garlic, minced
- 1 fresh lemon juice
- 1/4 cup olive oil
- Salt

DIRECTIONS

1. Add basil, vinegar, tomato paste, garlic, lemon juice, oil, and salt into the blender and blend until smooth.
2. Add eggplant, tomatoes, onion, squash, and zucchini into the instant pot.
3. Pour blended basil mixture over vegetables and stir well.
4. Seal pot with lid and cook on high for 10 minutes.
5. Once done, allow to release pressure naturally. Remove lid.
6. Stir well and serve.

NUTRITION: Calories 103 Fat 6.8 g Carbohydrates 10.6 g Sugar 6.1 g Protein 2.4 g Cholesterol 0 mg

261. Garlic Basil Zucchini

Preparation Time: 10 minutes

Cooking Time: 8 minutes

Servings: 4

INGREDIENTS

- 14 oz zucchini, sliced
- 1/4 cup fresh basil, chopped
- 1/2 tsp red pepper flakes

- 14 oz can tomatoes, chopped
- 1 tsp garlic, minced
- 1/2 onion, chopped
- 1/4 cup feta cheese, crumbled
- 1 tbsp olive oil
- Salt

DIRECTIONS

1. Add oil into the inner pot of instant pot and set the pot on sauté mode.
2. Add onion and garlic and sauté for 2 minutes.
3. Add remaining ingredients except feta cheese and stir well.
4. Seal pot with lid and cook on high for 6 minutes.
5. Once done, allow to release pressure naturally. Remove lid.
6. Top with feta cheese and serve.

NUTRITION: Calories 99 Fat 5.7 g Carbohydrates 10.4 g Sugar 6.1 g Protein 3.7 g Cholesterol 8 mg

262. Feta Green Beans

Preparation Time: 10 minutes

Cooking Time: 15 minutes

Servings: 4

INGREDIENTS

- 1 1/2 lbs green beans, trimmed
- 1/4 cup feta cheese, crumbled
- 28 oz can tomatoes, crushed
- 2 tsp oregano
- 1 tsp cumin
- 1/2 cup water
- 1 tbsp olive oil
- 1 tbsp garlic, minced
- 1 onion, chopped

- 1 lb baby potatoes, clean and cut into chunks
- Pepper
- Salt

DIRECTIONS

1. Add oil into the inner pot of instant pot and set the pot on sauté mode.
2. Add onion and garlic and sauté for 3-5 minutes.
3. Add remaining ingredients except feta cheese and stir well.
4. Seal pot with lid and cook on high for 10 minutes.
5. Once done, allow to release pressure naturally for 5 minutes then release remaining using quick release. Remove lid.
6. Top with feta cheese and serve.

NUTRITION: Calories 234 Fat 6.1 g Carbohydrates 40.7 g Sugar 10.7 g Protein 9.7 g Cholesterol 8 mg

263. Garlic Parmesan Artichokes

Preparation Time: 10 minutes

Cooking Time: 10 minutes

Servings: 4

INGREDIENTS

- 4 artichokes, wash, trim, and cut top
- 1/2 cup vegetable broth
- 1/4 cup parmesan cheese, grated
- 1 tbsp olive oil
- 2 tsp garlic, minced

Salt directions

1. Pour broth into the instant pot then place steamer rack in the pot.
2. Place artichoke steam side down on steamer rack into the pot.
3. Sprinkle garlic and grated cheese on top of artichokes and season with salt. Drizzle oil over artichokes.
4. Seal pot with lid and cook on high for 10 minutes.
5. Once done, release pressure using quick release. Remove lid.
6. Serve and enjoy.

NUTRITION: Calories 132 Fat 5.2 g Carbohydrates 17.8 g Sugar 1.7 g Protein 7.9 g Cholesterol 4 mg

264. Delicious Pepper Zucchini

Preparation Time: 10 minutes

Cooking Time: 10 minutes

Servings: 6

INGREDIENTS

- 1 zucchini, sliced
- 2 poblano peppers, sliced
- 1 tbsp sour cream
- 1/2 tsp ground cumin
- 1 yellow squash, sliced
- 1 tbsp garlic, minced
- 1/2 onion, sliced
- 1 tbsp olive oil
- Salt

DIRECTIONS

1. Add oil into the inner pot of instant pot and set the pot on sauté mode.

2. Add poblano peppers and sauté for 5 minutes
3. Add onion and garlic and sauté for 3 minutes.
4. Add remaining ingredients except for sour cream and stir well.
5. Seal pot with lid and cook on high for 2 minutes.
6. Once done, release pressure using quick release. Remove lid.
7. Add sour cream and stir well and serve.

NUTRITION: Calories 42 Fat 2.9 g Carbohydrates 4 g Sugar 1.7 g Protein 1 g Cholesterol 1 mg

265. Celery Carrot Brown Lentils

Preparation Time: 10 minutes

Cooking Time: 25 minutes

Servings: 6

- **INGREDIENTS**
- 2 cups dry brown lentils, rinsed and drained
- 2 1/2 cups vegetable stock
- 2 tomatoes, chopped
- 1/2 tsp red pepper flakes
- 1/2 tsp ground cinnamon
- 1 bay leaf
- 1 tbsp tomato paste
- 2 celery stalks, diced
- 2 carrots, grated
- 1 tbsp garlic, minced
- 2 onions, chopped
- 1/4 cup olive oil
- Pepper
- Salt

DIRECTIONS

1. Add oil into the inner pot of instant pot and set the pot on sauté mode.
2. Add celery, carrot, garlic, onion, pepper, and salt and sauté for 3 minutes.
3. Add remaining ingredients and stir everything well.
4. Seal pot with lid and cook on high for 22 minutes.
5. Once done, release pressure using quick release. Remove lid.
6. Stir well and serve.

NUTRITION: Calories 137 Fat 8.8 g Carbohydrates 12.3 g Sugar 4.7 g Protein 3.1 g Cholesterol 0 mg

266. **Lemon Artichokes**

- Preparation Time: 10 minutes
- Cooking Time: 20 minutes
- Servings: 4
- **INGREDIENTS**
- 4 artichokes, trim and cut the top
- 1/4 cup fresh lemon juice
- 2 cups vegetable stock
- 1 tsp lemon zest, grated
- Pepper
- Salt

DIRECTIONS

1. Pour the stock into the instant pot then place steamer rack in the pot.
2. Place artichoke steam side down on steamer rack into the pot.
3. Sprinkle lemon zest over artichokes. Season with pepper and salt.
4. Pour lemon juice over artichokes.
5. Seal pot with lid and cook on high for 20 minutes.

6. Once done, allow to release pressure naturally for 5 minutes then release remaining using quick release. Remove lid.
7. Serve and enjoy.

NUTRITION: Calories 83 Fat 0.4 g Carbohydrates 17.9 g Sugar 2.3 g Protein 5.6 g Cholesterol 0 mg

267. **Easy Chili Pepper Zucchinis**

Preparation Time: 10 minutes

Cooking Time: 10 minutes

Servings: 4

INGREDIENTS

- 4 zucchinis, cut into cubes
- 1/2 tsp red pepper flakes
- 1/2 tsp cayenne
- 1 tbsp chili powder
- 1/4 cup vegetable stock
- Salt

DIRECTIONS

1. Add all ingredients into the inner pot of instant pot and stir well.
2. Seal pot with lid and cook on high for 10 minutes.
3. Once done, allow to release pressure naturally for 10 minutes then release remaining using quick release. Remove lid.
4. Stir and serve.

NUTRITION: Calories 38 Fat 0.7 g Carbohydrates 8.8 g Sugar 3.6 g Protein 2.7 g Cholesterol 0 mg

268. <u>Delicious Okra</u>

Preparation Time: 10 minutes

Cooking Time: 10 minutes

Servings: 4

INGREDIENTS

- 2 cups okra, chopped
- 2 tbsp fresh dill, chopped
- 1 tbsp paprika
- 1 cup can tomato, crushed
- Pepper
- Salt

DIRECTIONS

1. Add all ingredients into the inner pot of instant pot and stir well.
2. Seal pot with lid and cook on high for 10 minutes.
3. Once done, allow to release pressure naturally for 5 minutes then release remaining using quick release. Remove lid.
4. Stir well and serve.

NUTRITION: Calories 37 Fat 0.5 g Carbohydrates 7.4 g Sugar 0.9 g Protein 2 g Cholesterol 0 mg

269. <u>Tomato Dill Cauliflower</u>

Preparation Time: 10 minutes

Cooking Time: 12 minutes

Servings: 4

INGREDIENTS

- 1 lb cauliflower florets, chopped

- 1 tbsp fresh dill, chopped
- 1/4 tsp Italian seasoning
- 1 tbsp vinegar
- 1 cup can tomatoes, crushed
- 1 cup vegetable stock
- 1 tsp garlic, minced
- Pepper
- Salt

DIRECTIONS

1. Add all ingredients except dill into the instant pot and stir well.
2. Seal pot with lid and cook on high for 12 minutes.
3. Once done, allow to release pressure naturally for 10 minutes then release remaining using quick release. Remove lid.
4. Garnish with dill and serve.

NUTRITION: Calories 47 Fat 0.3 g Carbohydrates 10 g Sugar 5 g Protein 3.1 g Cholesterol 0 mg

270. <u>Parsnips with Eggplant</u>

Preparation Time: 10 minutes

Cooking Time: 12 minutes

Servings: 4

INGREDIENTS

- 2 parsnips, sliced
- 1 cup can tomatoes, crushed
- 1/2 tsp ground cumin
- 1 tbsp paprika
- 1 tsp garlic, minced
- 1 eggplant, cut into chunks
- 1/4 tsp dried basil
- Pepper

- Salt

DIRECTIONS

Add all ingredients into the instant pot and stir well.

Seal pot with lid and cook on high for 12 minutes.

Once done, release pressure using quick release. Remove lid.

Stir and serve.

NUTRITION: Calories 98 0.7 g Carbohydrates 23 g Sugar 8.8 g Protein 2.8 g Cholesterol 0 mg

271.   **Easy Garlic Beans**

Preparation Time: 10 minutes

Cooking Time: 5 minutes

Servings: 4

INGREDIENTS

- 1 lb green beans, trimmed
- 1 1/2 cup vegetable stock
- 1 tsp garlic, minced
- 1 tbsp olive oil
- Pepper
- Salt

DIRECTIONS

1. Add all ingredients into the instant pot and stir well.
2. Seal pot with lid and cook on high for 5 minutes.
3. Once done, release pressure using quick release. Remove lid.
4. Stir and serve.

NUTRITION: Calories 69 Fat 3.7 g Carbohydrates 8.7 g Sugar 1.9 g Protein 2.3 g Cholesterol 0 mg

272.   **Eggplant with Olives**

Preparation Time: 10 minutes

Cooking Time: 12 minutes

Servings: 4

INGREDIENTS

- 4 cups eggplants, cut into cubes
- 1/2 cup vegetable stock
- 1 tsp chili powder
- 1 cup olives, pitted and sliced
- 1 onion, chopped
- 1 tbsp olive oil
- 1/4 cup grape tomatoes
- Pepper
- Salt

DIRECTIONS

1. Add oil into the inner pot of instant pot and set the pot on sauté mode.
2. Add onion and sauté for 2 minutes.
3. Add remaining ingredients and stir everything well.
4. Seal pot with lid and cook on high for 12 minutes.
5. Once done, allow to release pressure naturally for 10 minutes then release remaining using quick release. Remove lid.
6. Stir and serve.

NUTRITION: Calories 105 Fat 7.4 g Carbohydrates 10.4 g Sugar 4.1 g Protein 1.6 g Cholesterol 0 mg

273. Vegan Carrots & Broccoli

Preparation Time: 10 minutes

Cooking Time: 5 minutes

Servings: 6

INGREDIENTS

- 4 cups broccoli florets
- 2 carrots, peeled and sliced
- 1/4 cup water
- 1/2 lemon juice
- 1 tsp garlic, minced
- 1 tbsp olive oil
- 1/4 cup vegetable stock
- 1/4 tsp Italian seasoning
- Salt

DIRECTIONS

1. Add oil into the inner pot of instant pot and set the pot on sauté mode.
2. Add garlic and sauté for 30 seconds.
3. Add carrots and broccoli and cook for 2 minutes.
4. Add remaining ingredients and stir everything well.
5. Seal pot with lid and cook on high for 3 minutes.
6. Once done, release pressure using quick release. Remove lid.
7. Stir well and serve.

NUTRITION: Calories 51 Fat 2.6 g Carbohydrates 6.3 g Sugar 2.2 g Protein 2 g Cholesterol 0 mg

274. Zucchini Tomato Potato Ratatouille

Preparation Time: 10 minutes

Cooking Time: 10 minutes

Servings: 6

INGREDIENTS

- 1 1/2 lbs potatoes, cut into cubes
- 1/2 cup fresh basil
- 28 oz fire-roasted tomatoes, chopped
- 1 onion, chopped
- 4 mushrooms, sliced
- 1 bell pepper, diced
- 12 oz eggplant, diced
- 8 oz zucchini, diced
- 8 oz yellow squash, diced
- Pepper
- Salt

DIRECTIONS

1. Add all ingredients except basil into the instant pot and stir well.
2. Seal pot with lid and cook on high for 10 minutes.
3. Once done, release pressure using quick release. Remove lid.
4. Add basil and stir well and serve.

NUTRITION: Calories 175 Fat 1.9 g

POULTRY

275. Duck and Blackberries

Preparation time: 10 minutes

Cooking time: 25 minutes

Servings: 4

INGREDIENTS

- 4 duck breasts, boneless and skin scored
- 2 tablespoons balsamic vinegar
- Salt and black pepper to the taste
- 1 cup chicken stock
- 4 ounces blackberries
- ¼ cup chicken stock
- 2 tablespoons avocado oil

DIRECTIONS

1. between plates and serve.

NUTRITION: Calories 239, fat 10.5, fiber 10.2, carbs 21.1, protein 33.3

276. Ginger Ducated

- 2 big duck breasts, boneless and skin scored
- 2 tablespoons olive oil
- Salt and black pepper to the taste
- 1 tablespoon fish sauce
- 1 tablespoon lime juice
- 1 garlic clove, minced
- 1 Serrano chili, chopped
- 1 small shallot, sliced
- 1 cucumber, sliced
- 2 mangos, peeled and sliced
- ¼ cup oregano, chopped

DIRECTIONS

1. Heat up a pan with the oil over medium-high heat, add the duck breasts skin side down and cook for 5 minutes.
2. Add the orange zest, salt, pepper, fish sauce and the rest of the ingredients, bring to a simmer and cook over medium-low heat for 45 minutes.
3. Divide everything between plates and serve.

NUTRITION: Calories 297, fat 9.1, fiber 10.2, carbs 20.8, protein 16.5

277. Turkey and Cranberry Sauce

Preparation time: 10 minutes

Cooking time: 50 minutes

Servings: 4

INGREDIENTS

- 1 cup chicken stock
- 2 tablespoons avocado oil
- ½ cup cranberry sauce
- 1 big turkey breast, skinless, boneless and sliced
- 1 yellow onion, roughly chopped
- Salt and black pepper to the taste

DIRECTIONS

1. Heat up a pan with the avocado oil over medium-high heat, add the onion and sauté for 5 minutes.

2. Add the turkey and brown for 5 minutes more.
3. Add the rest of the ingredients, toss, introduce in the oven at 350 degrees F and cook for 40 minutes

NUTRITION: Calories 382, fat 12.6, fiber 9.6, carbs 26.6, protein 17.6

278. Sage Turkey Mix

Preparation time: 10 minutes

Cooking time: 40 minutes

Servings: 4

INGREDIENTS

- 1 big turkey breast, skinless, boneless and roughly cubed
- Juice of 1 lemon
- 2 tablespoons avocado oil
- 1 red onion, chopped
- 2 tablespoons sage, chopped
- 1 garlic clove, minced
- 1 cup chicken stock

DIRECTIONS

1. Heat up a pan with the avocado oil over medium-high heat, add the turkey and brown for 3 minutes on each side.
2. Add the rest of the ingredients, bring to a simmer and cook over medium heat for 35 minutes.
3. Divide the mix between plates and serve with a side dish.

NUTRITION: Calories 382, fat 12.6, fiber 9.6, carbs 16.6, protein 33.2

279. Turkey and Asparagus Mix

Preparation time: 10 minutes

Cooking time: 30 minutes

Servings: 4

INGREDIENTS

- 1 bunch asparagus, trimmed and halved
- 1 big turkey breast, skinless, boneless and cut into strips
- 1 teaspoon basil, dried
- 2 tablespoons olive oil
- A pinch of salt and black pepper
- ½ cup tomato sauce
- 1 tablespoon chives, chopped

DIRECTIONS

1. Heat up a pan with the oil over medium-high heat, add the turkey and brown for 4 minutes.
2. Add the asparagus and the rest of the ingredients except the chives, bring to a simmer and cook over medium heat for 25 minutes.
3. Add the chives, divide the mix between plates and serve.

NUTRITION: Calories 337, fat 21.2, fiber 10.2, carbs 21.4, protein 17.6

280. Herbed Almond Turkey

Preparation time: 10 minutes

Cooking time: 40 minutes

Servings: 4

INGREDIENTS

- 1 big turkey breast, skinless, boneless and cubed
- 1 tablespoon olive oil
- ½ cup chicken stock
- 1 tablespoon basil, chopped
- 1 tablespoon rosemary, chopped
- 1 tablespoon oregano, chopped
- 1 tablespoon parsley, chopped
- 3 garlic cloves, minced
- ½ cup almonds, toasted and chopped
- 3 cups tomatoes, chopped

DIRECTIONS

1. Heat up a pan with the oil over medium-high heat, add the turkey and the garlic and brown for 5 minutes.
2. Add the stock and the rest of the ingredients, bring to a simmer over medium heat and cook for 35 minutes.
3. Divide the mix between plates and serve.

NUTRITION: Calories 297, fat 11.2, fiber 9.2, carbs 19.4, protein 23.6

281. Thyme Chicken and Potatoes

Preparation time: 10 minutes

Cooking time: 50 minutes

Servings: 4

INGREDIENTS

- 1 tablespoon olive oil
- 4 garlic cloves, minced
- A pinch of salt and black pepper
- 2 teaspoons thyme, dried
- 12 small red potatoes, halved

- 2 pounds chicken breast, skinless, boneless and cubed
- 1 cup red onion, sliced
- ¾ cup chicken stock
- 2 tablespoons basil, chopped

DIRECTIONS

1. In a baking dish greased with the oil, add the potatoes, chicken and the rest of the ingredients, toss a bit, introduce in the oven and bake at 400 degrees F for 50 minutes.
2. Divide between plates and serve.

NUTRITION: Calories 281, fat 9.2, fiber 10.9, carbs 21.6, protein 13.6

282. Turkey, Artichokes and Asparagus

Preparation time: 10 minutes

Cooking time: 30 minutes

Servings: 4

INGREDIENTS

- 2 turkey breasts, boneless, skinless and halved
- 3 tablespoons olive oil
- 1 and ½ pounds asparagus, trimmed and halved
- 1 cup chicken stock
- A pinch of salt and black pepper
- 1 cup canned artichoke hearts, drained
- ¼ cup kalamata olives, pitted and sliced
- 1 shallot, chopped
- 3 garlic cloves, minced
- 3 tablespoons dill, chopped

DIRECTIONS

1. Heat up a pan with the oil over medium-high heat, add the turkey and the garlic and brown for 4 minutes on each side.
2. Add the asparagus, the stock and the rest of the ingredients except the dill, bring to a simmer and cook over medium heat for 20 minutes.
3. Add the dill, divide the mix between plates and serve.

NUTRITION: Calories 291, fat 16, fiber 10.3, carbs 22.8, protein 34.5

283. Lemony Turkey and Pine Nuts

Preparation time: 10 minutes

Cooking time: 30 minutes

Servings: 4

INGREDIENTS

- 2 turkey breasts, boneless, skinless and halved
- A pinch of salt and black pepper
- 2 tablespoons avocado oil
- Juice of 2 lemons
- 1 tablespoon rosemary, chopped
- 3 garlic cloves, minced
- ¼ cup pine nuts, chopped
- 1 cup chicken stock

DIRECTIONS

1. Heat up a pan with the oil over medium-high heat, add the garlic and the turkey and brown for 4 minutes on each side.

2. Add the rest of the ingredients, bring to a simmer and cook over medium heat for 20 minutes.
3. Divide the mix between plates and serve with a side salad.

NUTRITION: Calories 293, fat 12.4, fiber 9.3, carbs 17.8, protein 24.5

284. Yogurt Chicken and Red Onion Mix

Preparation time: 10 minutes

Cooking time: 30 minutes

Servings: 4

INGREDIENTS

- 2 pounds chicken breast, skinless, boneless and sliced
- 3 tablespoons olive oil
- ¼ cup Greek yogurt
- 2 garlic cloves, minced
- ½ teaspoon onion powder
- A pinch of salt and black pepper
- 4 red onions, sliced

DIRECTIONS

1. In a roasting pan, combine the chicken with the oil, the yogurt and the other ingredients, introduce in the oven at 375 degrees F and bake for 30 minutes.
2. Divide chicken mix between plates and serve hot.

NUTRITION: Calories 278, fat 15, fiber 9.2, carbs 15.1, protein 23.3

285. Chicken and Mint Sauce

Preparation time: 10 minutes

Cooking time: 30 minutes

Servings: 4

INGREDIENTS

- 2 and ½ tablespoons olive oil
- 2 pounds chicken breasts, skinless, boneless and halved
- 3 tablespoons garlic, minced
- 2 tablespoons lemon juice
- 1 tablespoon red wine vinegar
- 1/3 cup Greek yogurt
- 2 tablespoons mint, chopped
- A pinch of salt and black pepper

DIRECTIONS

1. In a blender, combine the garlic with the lemon juice and the other ingredients except the oil and the chicken and pulse well.
2. Heat up a pan with the oil over medium-high heat, add the chicken and brown for 3 minutes on each side.
3. Add the mint sauce, introduce in the oven and bake everything at 370 degrees F for 25 minutes.
4. Divide the mix between plates and serve.

NUTRITION: Calories 278, fat 12, fiber 11.2, carbs 18.1, protein 13.3

286. Oregano Turkey and Peppers

Preparation time: 10 minutes

Cooking time: 1 hour

Servings: 4

INGREDIENTS

- 2 red bell peppers, cut into strips
- 2 green bell peppers, cut into strips
- 1 red onion, chopped
- 4 garlic cloves, minced
- ½ cup black olives, pitted and sliced
- 2 cups chicken stock
- 1 big turkey breast, skinless, boneless and cut into strips
- 1 tablespoon oregano, chopped
- ½ cup cilantro, chopped

DIRECTIONS

1. In a baking pan, combine the peppers with the turkey and the rest of the ingredients, toss, introduce in the oven at 400 degrees F and roast for 1 hour.
2. Divide everything between plates and serve.

NUTRITION: Calories 229, fat 8.9, fiber 8.2, carbs 17.8, protein 33.6

287. Chicken and Mustard Sauce

Preparation time: 10 minutes

Cooking time: 26 minutes

Servings: 4

INGREDIENTS

- 1/3 cup mustard
- Salt and black pepper to the taste
- 1 red onion, chopped
- 1 tablespoon olive oil
- 1 and ½ cups chicken stock
- 4 chicken breasts, skinless, boneless and halved

• ¼ teaspoon oregano, dried

DIRECTIONS

1. Heat up a pan with the stock over medium heat, add the mustard, onion, salt, pepper and the oregano, whisk, bring to a simmer and cook for 8 minutes.
2. Heat up a pan with the oil over medium-high heat, add the chicken and brown for 3 minutes on each side.
3. Add the chicken to the pan with the sauce, toss, simmer everything for 12 minutes more, divide between plates and serve.

NUTRITION: Calories 247, fat 15.1, fiber 9.1, carbs 16.6, protein 26.1

288. Chicken and Sausage Mix

Preparation time: 10 minutes

Cooking time: 50 minutes

Servings: 4

INGREDIENTS

• 2 zucchinis, cubed
• 1 pound Italian sausage, cubed
• 2 tablespoons olive oil
• 1 red bell pepper, chopped
• 1 red onion, sliced
• 2 tablespoons garlic, minced
• 2 chicken breasts, boneless, skinless and halved
• Salt and black pepper to the taste
• ½ cup chicken stock
• 1 tablespoon balsamic vinegar

DIRECTIONS

1. Heat up a pan with half of the oil over medium-high heat, add the sausages, brown for 3 minutes on each side and transfer to a bowl.
2. Heat up the pan again with the rest of the oil over medium-high heat, add the chicken and brown for 4 minutes on each side.
3. Return the sausage, add the rest of the ingredients as well, bring to a simmer, introduce in the oven and bake at 400 degrees F for 30 minutes.
4. Divide everything between plates and serve.

NUTRITION: Calories 293, fat 13.1, fiber 8.1, carbs 16.6, protein 26.1

289. Coriander and Coconut Chicken

Preparation time: 10 minutes

Cooking time: 30 minutes

Servings: 4

INGREDIENTS

• 2 pounds chicken thighs, skinless, boneless and cubed
• 2 tablespoons olive oil
• Salt and black pepper to the taste
• 3 tablespoons coconut flesh, shredded
• 1 and ½ teaspoons orange extract
• 1 tablespoon ginger, grated
• ¼ cup orange juice
• 2 tablespoons coriander, chopped
• 1 cup chicken stock
• ¼ teaspoon red pepper flakes

DIRECTIONS

1. Heat up a pan with the oil over medium-high heat, add the chicken and brown for 4 minutes on each side.
2. Add salt, pepper and the rest of the ingredients, bring to a simmer and cook over medium heat for 20 minutes.
3. Divide the mix between plates and serve hot.

NUTRITION: Calories 297, fat 14.4, fiber 9.6, carbs 22, protein 25

290. Saffron Chicken Thighs and Green Beans

Preparation time: 10 minutes

Cooking time: 25 minutes

Servings: 4

INGREDIENTS

- 2 pounds chicken thighs, boneless and skinless
- 2 teaspoons saffron powder
- 1 pound green beans, trimmed and halved
- ½ cup Greek yogurt
- Salt and black pepper to the taste
- 1 tablespoon lime juice
- 1 tablespoon dill, chopped

DIRECTIONS

1. In a roasting pan, combine the chicken with the saffron, green beans and the rest of the ingredients, toss a bit, introduce in the oven and bake at 400 degrees F for 25 minutes.

2. Divide everything between plates and serve.

NUTRITION: Calories 274, fat 12.3, fiber 5.3, carbs 20.4, protein 14.3

291. Chicken and Olives Salsa

Preparation time: 10 minutes

Cooking time: 25 minutes

Servings: 4

INGREDIENTS

- 2 tablespoon avocado oil
- 4 chicken breast halves, skinless and boneless
- Salt and black pepper to the taste
- 1 tablespoon sweet paprika
- 1 red onion, chopped
- 1 tablespoon balsamic vinegar
- 2 tablespoons parsley, chopped
- 1 avocado, peeled, pitted and cubed
- 2 tablespoons black olives, pitted and chopped

DIRECTIONS

1. Heat up your grill over medium-high heat, add the chicken brushed with half of the oil and seasoned with paprika, salt and pepper, cook for 7 minutes on each side and divide between plates.
2. Meanwhile, in a bowl, mix the onion with the rest of the ingredients and the remaining oil, toss, add on top of the chicken and serve.

NUTRITION: Calories 289, fat 12.4, fiber 9.1, carbs 23.8, protein 14.3

292. Carrots and Tomatoes Chicken

Preparation time: 10 minutes

Cooking time: 1 hour and 10 minutes

Servings: 4

INGREDIENTS

- 2 pounds chicken breasts, skinless, boneless and halved
- Salt and black pepper to the taste
- 3 garlic cloves, minced
- 3 tablespoons avocado oil
- 2 shallots, chopped
- 4 carrots, sliced
- 3 tomatoes, chopped
- ¼ cup chicken stock
- 1 tablespoon Italian seasoning
- 1 tablespoon parsley, chopped

DIRECTIONS

1. Heat up a pan with the oil over medium-high heat, add the chicken, garlic, salt and pepper and brown for 3 minutes on each side.
2. Add the rest of the ingredients except the parsley, bring to a simmer and cook over medium-low heat for 40 minutes.
3. Add the parsley, divide the mix between plates and serve.

NUTRITION: Calories 309, fat 12.4, fiber 11.1, carbs 23.8, protein 15.3

293. Smoked and Hot Turkey Mix

Preparation time: 10 minutes

Cooking time: 40 minutes

Servings: 4

INGREDIENTS

- 1 red onion, sliced
- 1 big turkey breast, skinless, boneless and roughly cubed
- 1 tablespoon smoked paprika
- 2 chili peppers, chopped
- Salt and black pepper to the taste
- 2 tablespoons olive oil
- ½ cup chicken stock
- 1 tablespoon parsley, chopped
- 1 tablespoon cilantro, chopped

DIRECTIONS

1. Grease a roasting pan with the oil, add the turkey, onion, paprika and the rest of the ingredients, toss, introduce in the oven and bake at 425 degrees F for 40 minutes.
2. Divide the mix between plates and serve right away.

NUTRITION: Calories 310, fat 18.4, fiber 10.4, carbs 22.3, protein 33.4

294. Spicy Cumin Chicken

Preparation time: 10 minutes

Cooking time: 25 minutes

Servings: 4

INGREDIENTS

- 2 teaspoons chili powder
- 2 and ½ tablespoons olive oil
- Salt and black pepper to the taste
- 1 and ½ teaspoons garlic powder
- 1 tablespoon smoked paprika
- ½ cup chicken stock
- 1 pound chicken breasts, skinless, boneless and halved
- 2 teaspoons sherry vinegar
- 2 teaspoons hot sauce
- 2 teaspoons cumin, ground
- ½ cup black olives, pitted and sliced

DIRECTIONS

1. Heat up a pan with the oil over medium-high heat, add the chicken and brown for 3 minutes on each side.
2. Add the chili powder, salt, pepper, garlic powder and paprika, toss and cook for 4 minutes more.
3. Add the rest of the ingredients, toss, bring to a simmer and cook over medium heat for 15 minutes more.
4. Divide the mix between plates and serve.

NUTRITION: Calories 230, fat 18.4, fiber 9.4, carbs 15.3, protein 13.4

295. Chicken with Artichokes and Beans

Preparation time: 10 minutes

Cooking time: 40 minutes

Servings: 4

INGREDIENTS

- 2 tablespoons olive oil

- 2 chicken breasts, skinless, boneless and halved
- Zest of 1 lemon, grated
- 3 garlic cloves, crushed
- Juice of 1 lemon
- Salt and black pepper to the taste
- 1 tablespoon thyme, chopped
- 6 ounces canned artichokes hearts, drained
- 1 cup canned fava beans, drained and rinsed
- 1 cup chicken stock
- A pinch of cayenne pepper
- Salt and black pepper to the taste

DIRECTIONS

1. Heat up a pan with the oil over medium-high heat, add chicken and brown for 5 minutes.
2. Add lemon juice, lemon zest, salt, pepper and the rest of the ingredients, bring to a simmer and cook over medium heat for 35 minutes.
3. Divide the mix between plates and serve right away.

NUTRITION: Calories 291, fat 14.9, fiber 10.5, carbs 23.8, protein 24.2

296. Chicken and Olives Tapenade

Preparation time: 10 minutes

Cooking time: 25 minutes

Servings: 4

INGREDIENTS

- 2 chicken breasts, boneless, skinless and halved
- 1 cup black olives, pitted

- ½ cup olive oil
- Salt and black pepper to the taste
- ½ cup mixed parsley, chopped
- ½ cup rosemary, chopped
- Salt and black pepper to the taste
- 4 garlic cloves, minced
- Juice of ½ lime

DIRECTIONS

1. In a blender, combine the olives with half of the oil and the rest of the ingredients except the chicken and pulse well.
2. Heat up a pan with the rest of the oil over medium-high heat, add the chicken and brown for 4 minutes on each side.
3. Add the olives mix, and cook for 20 minutes more tossing often.

NUTRITION: Calories 291, fat 12.9, fiber 8.5, carbs 15.8, protein 34.2

297. Spiced Chicken Meatballs

Preparation time: 10 minutes

Cooking time: 20 minutes

Servings: 4

INGREDIENTS

- 1 pound chicken meat, ground
- 1 tablespoon pine nuts, toasted and chopped
- 1 egg, whisked
- 2 teaspoons turmeric powder
- 2 garlic cloves, minced
- Salt and black pepper to the taste
- 1 and ¼ cups heavy cream
- 2 tablespoons olive oil
- ¼ cup parsley, chopped

- 1 tablespoon chives, chopped

DIRECTIONS

1. In a bowl, combine the chicken with the pine nuts and the rest of the ingredients except the oil and the cream, stir well and shape medium meatballs out of this mix.
2. Heat up a pan with the oil over medium-high heat, add the meatballs and cook them for 4 minutes on each side.
3. Add the cream, toss gently, cook everything over medium heat for 10 minutes more, divide between plates and serve.

NUTRITION: Calories 283, fat 9.2, fiber 12.8, carbs 24.4, protein 34.5

298. Sesame Turkey Mix

Preparation time: 10 minutes

Cooking time: 25 minutes

Servings: 4

INGREDIENTS

- 2 tablespoons avocado oil
- 1 and ¼ cups chicken stock
- 1 tablespoons sesame seeds, toasted
- Salt and black pepper to the taste
- 1 big turkey breast, skinless, boneless and sliced
- ¼ cup parsley, chopped
- 4 ounces feta cheese, crumbled
- ¼ cup red onion, chopped
- 1 tablespoon lemon juice

DIRECTIONS

1. Heat up a pan with the oil over medium-high heat, add the meat and brown for 4 minutes on each side.
2. Add the rest of the ingredients except the cheese and the sesame seeds, bring everything to a simmer and cook over medium heat for 15 minutes.
3. Add the cheese, toss, divide the mix between plates, sprinkle the sesame seeds on top and serve.

NUTRITION: Calories 283, fat 13.2, fiber 6.8, carbs 19.4, protein 24.5

299. Cardamom Chicken and Apricot Sauce

Preparation time: 10 minutes

Cooking time: 7 hours

Servings: 4

INGREDIENTS

- Juice of ½ lemon
- Zest of ½ lemon, grated
- 2 teaspoons cardamom, ground
- Salt and black pepper to the taste
- 2 chicken breasts, skinless, boneless and halved
- 2 tablespoons olive oil
- 2 spring onions, chopped
- 2 tablespoons tomato paste
- 2 garlic cloves, minced
- 1 cup apricot juice
- ½ cup chicken stock
- ¼ cup cilantro, chopped

DIRECTIONS

1. In your slow cooker, combine the chicken with the lemon juice, lemon zest and the other ingredients except the cilantro, toss, put the lid on and cook on Low for 7 hours.
2. Divide the mix between plates, sprinkle the cilantro on top and serve.

NUTRITION: Calories 323, fat 12, fiber 11, carbs 23.8, protein 16.4

MEAT

300. Moist Shredded Beef

Preparation Time: 10 minutes

Cooking Time: 20 minutes

Servings: 8

INGREDIENTS

- 2 lbs beef chuck roast, cut into chunks
- 1/2 tbsp dried red pepper
- 1 tbsp Italian seasoning
- 1 tbsp garlic, minced
- 2 tbsp vinegar
- 14 oz can fire-roasted tomatoes
- 1/2 cup bell pepper, chopped
- 1/2 cup carrots, chopped
- 1 cup onion, chopped
- 1 tsp salt

DIRECTIONS

1. Add all ingredients into the inner pot of instant pot and set the pot on sauté mode.
2. Seal pot with lid and cook on high for 20 minutes.
3. Once done, release pressure using quick release. Remove lid.
4. Shred the meat using a fork.
5. Stir well and serve.

NUTRITION: Calories 456 Fat 32.7 g Carbohydrates 7.7 g Sugar 4.1 g Protein 31 g Cholesterol 118 mg

301. Hearty Beef Ragu

Preparation Time: 10 minutes

Cooking Time: 50 minutes

Servings: 4

INGREDIENTS

- 1 1/2 lbs beef steak, diced
- 1 1/2 cup beef stock
- 1 tbsp coconut amino
- 14 oz can tomatoes, chopped
- 1/2 tsp ground cinnamon
- 1 tsp dried oregano
- 1 tsp dried thyme
- 1 tsp dried basil
- 1 tsp paprika
- 1 bay leaf
- 1 tbsp garlic, chopped
- 1/2 tsp cayenne pepper
- 1 celery stick, diced
- 1 carrot, diced
- 1 onion, diced
- 2 tbsp olive oil
- 1/4 tsp pepper
- 1 1/2 tsp sea salt

DIRECTIONS

1. Add oil into the instant pot and set the pot on sauté mode.
2. Add celery, carrots, onion, and salt and sauté for 5 minutes.
3. Add meat and remaining ingredients and stir everything well.
4. Seal pot with lid and cook on high for 30 minutes.
5. Once done, allow to release pressure naturally for 10 minutes then release

remaining using quick release. Remove lid.

6. Shred meat using a fork. Set pot on sauté mode and cook for 10 minutes. Stir every 2-3 minutes.
7. Serve and enjoy.

NUTRITION: Calories 435 Fat 18.1 g Carbohydrates 12.3 g Sugar 5.5 g Protein 54.4 g Cholesterol 152 mg

302. Dill Beef Brisket

Preparation Time: 10 minutes

Cooking Time: 50 minutes

Servings: 4

INGREDIENTS

- 2 1/2 lbs beef brisket, cut into cubes
- 2 1/2 cups beef stock
- 2 tbsp dill, chopped
- 1 celery stalk, chopped
- 1 onion, sliced
- 1 tbsp garlic, minced
- Pepper
- Salt

DIRECTIONS

1. Add all ingredients into the inner pot of instant pot and stir well.
2. Seal pot with lid and cook on high for 50 minutes.
3. Once done, allow to release pressure naturally for 10 minutes then release remaining using quick release. Remove lid.
4. Serve and enjoy.

NUTRITION: Calories 556 Fat 18.1 g Carbohydrates 4.3 g Sugar 1.3 g Protein 88.5 g Cholesterol 253 mg

303. Tasty Beef Stew

Preparation Time: 10 minutes

Cooking Time: 30 minutes

Servings: 4

INGREDIENTS

- 2 1/2 lbs beef roast, cut into chunks
- 1 cup beef broth
- 1/2 cup balsamic vinegar
- 1 tbsp honey
- 1/2 tsp red pepper flakes
- 1 tbsp garlic, minced
- Pepper
- Salt

DIRECTIONS

1. Add all ingredients into the inner pot of instant pot and stir well.
2. Seal pot with lid and cook on high for 30 minutes.
3. Once done, allow to release pressure naturally. Remove lid.
4. Stir well and serve.

NUTRITION: Calories 562 Fat 18.1 g Carbohydrates 5.7 g Sugar 4.6 g Protein 87.4 g Cholesterol 253 mg Meatloaf Preparation Time: 10 minutes Cooking Time: 35 minutes Servings: 6

INGREDIENTS

- 2 lbs ground beef
- 2 eggs, lightly beaten
- 1/4 tsp dried basil

- 3 tbsp olive oil
- 1/2 tsp dried sage
- 1 1/2 tsp dried parsley
- 1 tsp oregano
- 2 tsp thyme
- 1 tsp rosemary
- Pepper
- Salt

DIRECTIONS

1. Pour 1 1/2 cups of water into the instant pot then place the trivet in the pot.
2. Spray loaf pan with cooking spray.
3. Add all ingredients into the mixing bowl and mix until well combined.
4. Transfer meat mixture into the prepared loaf pan and place loaf pan on top of the trivet in the pot.
5. Seal pot with lid and cook on high for 35 minutes.
6. Once done, allow to release pressure naturally for 10 minutes then release remaining using quick release. Remove lid.
7. Serve and enjoy.

NUTRITION: Calories 365 Fat 18 g Carbohydrates 0.7 g Sugar 0.1 g Protein 47.8 g Cholesterol 190 mg

304. Flavorful Beef Bourguignon

Preparation Time: 10 minutes

Cooking Time: 20 minutes

Servings: 4

INGREDIENTS

- 1 1/2 lbs beef chuck roast, cut into chunks

- 2/3 cup beef stock
- 2 tbsp fresh thyme
- 1 bay leaf
- 1 tsp garlic, minced
- 8 oz mushrooms, sliced
- 2 tbsp tomato paste
- 2/3 cup dry red wine
- 1 onion, sliced
- 4 carrots, cut into chunks
- 1 tbsp olive oil
- Pepper
- Salt

DIRECTIONS

1. Add oil into the instant pot and set the pot on sauté mode.
2. Add meat and sauté until brown. Add onion and sauté until softened.
3. Add remaining ingredients and stir well.
4. Seal pot with lid and cook on high for 12 minutes.
5. Once done, allow to release pressure naturally. Remove lid.
6. Stir well and serve.

NUTRITION: Calories 744 Fat 51.3 g Carbohydrates 14.5 g Sugar 6.5 g Protein 48.1 g Cholesterol 175 mg

305. Delicious Beef Chili

Preparation Time: 10 minutes

Cooking Time: 35 minutes

Servings: 8

INGREDIENTS

- 2 lbs ground beef
- 1 tsp olive oil
- 1 tsp garlic, minced

- 1 small onion, chopped
- 2 tbsp chili powder
- 1 tsp oregano
- 1/2 tsp thyme
- 28 oz can tomatoes, crushed
- 2 cups beef stock
- 2 carrots, chopped
- 3 sweet potatoes, peeled and cubed
- Pepper
- Salt

DIRECTIONS

1. Add oil into the instant pot and set the pot on sauté mode.
2. Add meat and cook until brown.
3. Add remaining ingredients and stir well.
4. Seal pot with lid and cook on high for 35 minutes.
5. Once done, allow to release pressure naturally. Remove lid.
6. Stir well and serve.

NUTRITION: Calories 302 Fat 8.2 g Carbohydrates 19.2 g Sugar 4.8 g Protein 37.1 g Cholesterol 101 mg

306. Rosemary Creamy Beef

Preparation Time: 10 minutes

Cooking Time: 40 minutes

Servings: 4

INGREDIENTS

- 2 lbs beef stew meat, cubed
- 2 tbsp fresh parsley, chopped
- 1 tsp garlic, minced
- 1/2 tsp dried rosemary
- 1 tsp chili powder
- 1 cup beef stock

- 1 cup heavy cream
- 1 onion, chopped
- 1 tbsp olive oil
- Pepper
- Salt

DIRECTIONS

1. Add oil into the instant pot and set the pot on sauté mode.
2. Add rosemary, garlic, onion, and chili powder and sauté for 5 minutes.
3. Add meat and cook for 5 minutes.
4. Add remaining ingredients and stir well.
5. Seal pot with lid and cook on high for 30 minutes.
6. Once done, allow to release pressure naturally for 10 minutes then release remaining using quick release. Remove lid.
7. Serve and enjoy.

NUTRITION: Calories 574 Fat 29 g Carbohydrates 4.3 g Sugar 1.3 g Protein 70.6 g Cholesterol 244 mg

307. Spicy Beef Chili Verde

Preparation Time: 10 minutes

Cooking Time: 23 minutes

Servings: 2

INGREDIENTS

- 1/2 lb beef stew meat, cut into cubes
- 1/4 tsp chili powder
- 1 tbsp olive oil
- 1 cup chicken broth
- 1 Serrano pepper, chopped
- 1 tsp garlic, minced
- 1 small onion, chopped

- 1/4 cup grape tomatoes, chopped
- 1/4 cup tomatillos, chopped
- Pepper
- Salt

DIRECTIONS

1. Add oil into the instant pot and set the pot on sauté mode.
2. Add garlic and onion and sauté for 3 minutes.
3. Add remaining ingredients and stir well.
4. Seal pot with lid and cook on high for 20 minutes.
5. Once done, allow to release pressure naturally. Remove lid.
6. Stir well and serve.

NUTRITION: Calories 317 Fat 15.1 g Carbohydrates 6.4 g Sugar 2.6 g Protein 37.8 g Cholesterol 101 mg

308. Carrot Mushroom Beef Roast

Preparation Time: 10 minutes

Cooking Time: 40 minutes

Servings: 4

INGREDIENTS

- 1 1/2 lbs beef roast
- 1 tsp paprika
- 1/4 tsp dried rosemary
- 1 tsp garlic, minced
- 1/2 lb mushrooms, sliced
- 1/2 cup chicken stock
- 2 carrots, sliced
- Pepper
- Salt

DIRECTIONS

1. Add all ingredients into the inner pot of instant pot and stir well.
2. Seal pot with lid and cook on high for 40 minutes.
3. Once done, allow to release pressure naturally for 10 minutes then release remaining using quick release. Remove lid.
4. Slice and serve.

NUTRITION: Calories 345 Fat 10.9 g Carbohydrates 5.6 g Sugar 2.6 g Protein 53.8 g Cholesterol 152 mg

309. Italian Beef Roast

Preparation Time: 10 minutes

Cooking Time: 50 minutes

Servings: 6

INGREDIENTS

- 2 1/2 lbs beef roast, cut into chunks
- 1 cup chicken broth
- 1 cup red wine
- 2 tbsp Italian seasoning
- 2 tbsp olive oil
- 1 bell pepper, chopped
- 2 celery stalks, chopped
- 1 tsp garlic, minced
- 1 onion, sliced
- Pepper
- Salt

DIRECTIONS

1. Add oil into the instant pot and set the pot on sauté mode.
2. Add the meat into the pot and sauté until brown.

3. Add onion, bell pepper, and celery and sauté for 5 minutes.
4. Add remaining ingredients and stir well.
5. Seal pot with lid and cook on high for 40 minutes.
6. Once done, allow to release pressure naturally. Remove lid.
7. Stir well and serve.

NUTRITION: Calories 460 Fat 18.2 g Carbohydrates 5.3 g Sugar 2.7 g Protein 58.7 g Cholesterol 172 mg

310. Thyme Beef Round Roast

Preparation Time: 10 minutes

Cooking Time: 55 minutes

Servings: 8

INGREDIENTS

- 4 lbs beef bottom round roast, cut into pieces
- 2 tbsp honey
- 5 fresh thyme sprigs
- 2 cups red wine
- 1 lb carrots, cut into chunks
- 2 cups chicken broth
- 6 garlic cloves, smashed
- 1 onion, diced
- 1/4 cup olive oil
- 2 lbs potatoes, peeled and cut into chunks
- Pepper
- Salt

DIRECTIONS

1. Add all ingredients except carrots and potatoes into the instant pot.

2. Seal pot with lid and cook on high for 45 minutes.
3. Once done, release pressure using quick release. Remove lid.
4. Add carrots and potatoes and stir well.
5. Seal pot again with lid and cook on high for 10 minutes.
6. Once done, allow to release pressure naturally. Remove lid.
7. Stir well and serve.

NUTRITION: Calories 648 Fat 21.7 g Carbohydrates 33.3 g Sugar 9.7 g Protein 67.1 g Cholesterol 200 mg

311. Jalapeno Beef Chili

Preparation Time: 10 minutes

Cooking Time: 40 minutes

Servings: 8

INGREDIENTS

- 1 lb ground beef
- 1 tsp garlic powder
- 1 jalapeno pepper, chopped
- 1 tbsp ground cumin
- 1 tbsp chili powder
- 1 lb ground pork
- 4 tomatillos, chopped
- 1/2 onion, chopped
- 5 oz tomato paste
- Pepper
- Salt

DIRECTIONS

1. Add oil into the instant pot and set the pot on sauté mode.
2. Add beef and pork and cook until brown.

3. Add remaining ingredients and stir well.
4. Seal pot with lid and cook on high for 35 minutes.
5. Once done, allow to release pressure naturally. Remove lid.
6. Stir well and serve.

NUTRITION: Calories 217 Fat 6.1 g Carbohydrates 6.2 g Sugar 2.7 g Protein 33.4 g Cholesterol 92 mg

312. Beef with Tomatoes

Preparation Time: 10 minutes

Cooking Time: 40 minutes

Servings: 4

INGREDIENTS

- 2 lb beef roast, sliced
- 1 tbsp chives, chopped
- 1 tsp garlic, minced
- 1/2 tsp chili powder
- 2 tbsp olive oil
- 1 onion, chopped
- 1 cup beef stock
- 1 tbsp oregano, chopped
- 1 cup tomatoes, chopped
- Pepper
- Salt

DIRECTIONS

1. Add oil into the instant pot and set the pot on sauté mode.
2. Add garlic, onion, and chili powder and sauté for 5 minutes.
3. Add meat and cook for 5 minutes.
4. Add remaining ingredients and stir well.

5. Seal pot with lid and cook on high for 30 minutes.
6. Once done, allow to release pressure naturally for 10 minutes then release remaining using quick release. Remove lid.
7. Stir well and serve.

NUTRITION: Calories 511 Fat 21.6 g Carbohydrates 5.6 g Sugar 2.5 g Protein 70.4 g Cholesterol 203 mg

313. Tasty Beef Goulash

Preparation Time: 10 minutes

Cooking Time: 30 minutes

Servings: 2

INGREDIENTS

- 1/2 lb beef stew meat, cubed
- 1 tbsp olive oil
- 1/2 onion, chopped
- 1/2 cup sun-dried tomatoes, chopped
- 1/4 zucchini, chopped
- 1/2 cabbage, sliced
- 1 1/2 tbsp olive oil
- 2 cups chicken broth
- Pepper
- Salt

DIRECTIONS

1. Add oil into the instant pot and set the pot on sauté mode.
2. Add onion and sauté for 3-5 minutes.
3. Add tomatoes and cook for 5 minutes.
4. Add remaining ingredients and stir well.
5. Seal pot with lid and cook on high for 20 minutes.

6. Once done, allow to release pressure naturally for 10 minutes then release remaining using quick release. Remove lid.
7. Stir well and serve.

NUTRITION: Calories 389 Fat 15.8 g Carbohydrates 19.3 g Sugar 10.7 g Protein 43.2 g Cholesterol 101 mg

314. <u>**Beef & Beans**</u>

Preparation Time: 10 minutes

Cooking Time: 30 minutes

Servings: 4

INGREDIENTS

- 1 1/2 lbs beef, cubed
- 8 oz can tomatoes, chopped
- 8 oz red beans, soaked overnight and rinsed
- 1 tsp garlic, minced
- 1 1/2 cups beef stock
- 1/2 tsp chili powder
- 1 tbsp paprika
- 2 tbsp olive oil
- 1 onion, chopped
- Pepper
- Salt

DIRECTIONS

1. Add oil into the instant pot and set the pot on sauté mode.
2. Add meat and cook for 5 minutes.
3. Add garlic and onion and sauté for 5 minutes.
4. Add remaining ingredients and stir well.
5. Seal pot with lid and cook on high for 25 minutes.

6. Once done, allow to release pressure naturally. Remove lid.
7. Stir well and serve.

NUTRITION: Calories 604 Fat 18.7 g Carbohydrates 41.6 g Sugar 4.5 g Protein 66.6 g Cholesterol 152 mg

315. <u>**Delicious Ground Beef**</u>

Preparation Time: 10 minutes

Cooking Time: 10 minutes

Servings: 4

INGREDIENTS

- 1 lb ground beef
- 1 tbsp olive oil
- 2 tbsp tomato paste
- 1 cup chicken broth
- 12 oz cheddar cheese, shredded
- 1 tbsp Italian seasoning
- Pepper
- Salt

DIRECTIONS

1. Add oil into the instant pot and set the pot on sauté mode.
2. Add meat and cook until browned.
3. Add remaining ingredients except for cheese and stir well.
4. Seal pot with lid and cook on high for 7 minutes.
5. Once done, release pressure using quick release. Remove lid.
6. Add cheese and stir well and cook on sauté mode until cheese is melted.
7. Serve and enjoy.

NUTRITION: Calories 610 Fat 40.2 g Carbohydrates 3.2 g Sugar 1.9 g Protein 57.2 g Cholesterol 193 mg

NUTRITION: Calories 409 Fat 8.3 g Carbohydrates 36.3 g Sugar 4.2 g Protein 46.6 g Cholesterol 101 mg

316. <u>Bean Beef Chili</u>

Preparation Time: 10 minutes

Cooking Time: 40 minutes

Servings: 4

INGREDIENTS

1 lb ground beef

1/2 onion, diced

1/2 jalapeno pepper, minced

- 1 tsp chili powder
- 1/2 bell pepper, chopped
- 1 tsp garlic, chopped
- 1 cup chicken broth
- 14 oz can black beans, rinsed and drained
- 14 oz can red beans, rinsed and drained
- Pepper
- Salt

DIRECTIONS

1. Set instant pot on sauté mode.
2. Add meat and sauté until brown.
3. Add remaining ingredients and stir well.
4. Seal pot with lid and cook on high for 35 minutes.
5. Once done, release pressure using quick release. Remove lid.
6. Stir well and serve.

317. <u>Garlic Caper Beef Roast</u>

Preparation Time: 10 minutes

Cooking Time: 40 minutes

Servings: 4

INGREDIENTS

- 2 lbs beef roast, cubed
- 1 tbsp fresh parsley, chopped
- 1 tbsp capers, chopped
- 1 tbsp garlic, minced
- 1 cup chicken stock
- 1/2 tsp dried rosemary
- 1/2 tsp ground cumin
- 1 onion, chopped
- 1 tbsp olive oil
- Pepper
- Salt

DIRECTIONS

1. Add oil into the instant pot and set the pot on sauté mode.
2. Add garlic and onion and sauté for 5 minutes.
3. Add meat and cook until brown.
4. Add remaining ingredients and stir well.
5. Seal pot with lid and cook on high for 30 minutes.
6. Once done, allow to release pressure naturally. Remove lid.
7. Stir well and serve.

NUTRITION: Calories 470 Fat 17.9 g Carbohydrates 3.9 g Sugar 1.4 g Protein 69.5 g Cholesterol 203 mg

318. Cauliflower Tomato Beef

Preparation Time: 10 minutes

Cooking Time: 25 minutes

Servings: 2

INGREDIENTS

- 1/2 lb beef stew meat, chopped
- 1 tsp paprika
- 1 tbsp balsamic vinegar
- 1 celery stalk, chopped
- 1/4 cup grape tomatoes, chopped
- 1 onion, chopped
- 1 tbsp olive oil
- 1/4 cup cauliflower, chopped
- Pepper
- Salt

DIRECTIONS

1. Add oil into the instant pot and set the pot on sauté mode.
2. Add meat and sauté for 5 minutes.
3. Add remaining ingredients and stir well.
4. Seal pot with lid and cook on high for 20 minutes.
5. Once done, allow to release pressure naturally. Remove lid.
6. Stir and serve.

NUTRITION: Calories 306 Fat 14.3 g Carbohydrates 7.6 g Sugar 3.5 g Protein 35.7 g Cholesterol 101 mg

319. Artichoke Beef Roast

Preparation Time: 10 minutes

Cooking Time: 45 minutes

Servings: 6

INGREDIENTS

- 2 lbs beef roast, cubed
- 1 tbsp garlic, minced
- 1 onion, chopped
- 1/2 tsp paprika
- 1 tbsp parsley, chopped
- 2 tomatoes, chopped
- 1 tbsp capers, chopped
- 10 oz can artichokes, drained and chopped
- 2 cups chicken stock
- 1 tbsp olive oil
- Pepper
- Salt

DIRECTIONS

1. Add oil into the instant pot and set the pot on sauté mode.
2. Add garlic and onion and sauté for 5 minutes.
3. Add meat and cook until brown.
4. Add remaining ingredients and stir well.
5. Seal pot with lid and cook on high for 35 minutes.
6. Once done, allow to release pressure naturally. Remove lid.
7. Serve and enjoy.

NUTRITION: Calories 344 Fat 12.2 g Carbohydrates 9.2 g Sugar 2.6 g Protein 48.4 g Cholesterol 135 mg

320. Italian Beef

Preparation Time: 10 minutes

Cooking Time: 35 minutes

Servings: 4

INGREDIENTS

- 1 lb ground beef
- 1 tbsp olive oil
- 1/2 cup mozzarella cheese, shredded
- 1/2 cup tomato puree
- 1 tsp basil
- 1 tsp oregano
- 1/2 onion, chopped
- 1 carrot, chopped
- 14 oz can tomatoes, diced
- Pepper
- Salt

DIRECTIONS

1. Add oil into the instant pot and set the pot on sauté mode.
2. Add onion and sauté for 2 minutes.
3. Add meat and sauté until browned.
4. Add remaining ingredients except for cheese and stir well.
5. Seal pot with lid and cook on high for 35 minutes.
6. Once done, release pressure using quick release. Remove lid.
7. Add cheese and stir well and cook on sauté mode until cheese is melted.
8. Serve and enjoy.

NUTRITION: Calories 297 Fat 11.3 g Carbohydrates 11.1 g Sugar 6.2 g Protein 37.1 g Cholesterol 103 mg

321. Greek Chuck Roast

Preparation Time: 10 minutes

Cooking Time: 35 minutes

Servings: 6

INGREDIENTS

- 3 lbs beef chuck roast, boneless and cut into chunks
- 1/2 tsp dried basil
- 1 tsp oregano, chopped
- 1 small onion, chopped
- 1 cup tomatoes, diced
- 2 cups chicken broth
- 1 tbsp olive oil
- 1 tbsp garlic, minced
- Pepper
- Salt

DIRECTIONS

1. Add oil into the instant pot and set the pot on sauté mode.
2. Add onion and garlic and sauté for 3-5 minutes.
3. Add meat and sauté for 5 minutes.
4. Add remaining ingredients and stir well.
5. Seal pot with lid and cook on high for 25 minutes.
6. Once done, allow to release pressure naturally. Remove lid.
7. Serve and enjoy.

NUTRITION: Calories 869 Fat 66 g Carbohydrates 3.2 g Sugar 1.5 g Protein 61.5 g Cholesterol 234 mg

322. Beanless Beef Chili

Preparation Time: 10 minutes

Cooking Time: 20 minutes

Servings: 4

INGREDIENTS

- 1 lb ground beef
- 1/2 tsp dried rosemary
- 1/2 tsp paprika

- 1 tsp garlic powder
- 1/2 tsp chili powder
- 1/2 cup chicken broth
- 1 cup heavy cream
- 1 tbsp olive oil
- 1 tsp garlic, minced
- 1 small onion, chopped
- 1 bell pepper, chopped
- 2 cups tomatoes, diced
- Pepper
- Salt

DIRECTIONS

1. Add oil into the instant pot and set the pot on sauté mode.
2. Add meat, bell pepper, and onion and sauté for 5 minutes.
3. Add remaining ingredients except for heavy cream and stir well.
4. Seal pot with lid and cook on high for 5 minutes.
5. Once done, release pressure using quick release. Remove lid.
6. Add heavy cream and stir well and cook on sauté mode for 10 minutes.
7. Serve and enjoy.

NUTRITION: Calories 387 Fat 22.2 g Carbohydrates 9.5 g Sugar 5 g Protein 37.2 g Cholesterol 142 mg

323. Sage Tomato Beef

Preparation Time: 10 minutes

Cooking Time: 40 minutes

Servings: 4

INGREDIENTS

- 2 lbs beef stew meat, cubed
- 1/4 cup tomato paste

- 1 tsp garlic, minced
- 2 cups chicken stock
- 1 onion, chopped
- 2 tbsp olive oil
- 1 tbsp sage, chopped
- Pepper
- Salt

DIRECTIONS

1. Add oil into the instant pot and set the pot on sauté mode.
2. Add garlic and onion and sauté for 5 minutes.
3. Add meat and sauté for 5 minutes.
4. Add remaining ingredients and stir well.
5. Seal pot with lid and cook on high for 30 minutes.
6. Once done, allow to release pressure naturally. Remove lid.
7. Serve and enjoy.

NUTRITION: Calories 515 Fat 21.5 g Carbohydrates 7 g Sugar 3.6 g Protein 70 g Cholesterol 203 mg

324. Rosemary Beef Eggplant

Preparation Time: 10 minutes

Cooking Time: 30 minutes

Servings: 4

INGREDIENTS

- 1 lb beef stew meat, cubed
- 2 tbsp green onion, chopped
- 1/4 tsp red pepper flakes
- 1/2 tsp dried rosemary
- 1/2 tsp paprika
- 1 cup chicken stock
- 1 onion, chopped

- 1 eggplant, cubed
- 2 tbsp olive oil
- Pepper
- Salt

DIRECTIONS

1. Add oil into the instant pot and set the pot on sauté mode.
2. Add meat and onion and sauté for 5 minutes.
3. Add remaining ingredients and stir well.
4. Seal pot with lid and cook on high for 25 minutes.
5. Once done, allow to release pressure naturally. Remove lid.
6. Serve and enjoy.

NUTRITION: Calories 315 Fat 14.5 g Carbohydrates 10 gSugar 4.9 g Protein 36.1 g Cholesterol 101 mg

325. Lemon Basil Beef

Preparation Time: 10 minutes

Cooking Time: 35 minutes

Servings: 4

INGREDIENTS

- 1 1/2 lb beef stew meat, cut into cubes
- 1/2 cup fresh basil, chopped
- 1/2 tsp dried thyme
- 2 cups chicken stock
- 1 tsp garlic, minced
- 2 tbsp lemon juice
- 1 onion, chopped
- 2 tbsp olive oil
- Pepper
- Salt

DIRECTIONS

1. Add oil into the instant pot and set the pot on sauté mode.
2. Add meat, garlic, and onion and sauté for 5 minutes.
3. Add remaining ingredients and stir well.
4. Seal pot with lid and cook on high for 30 minutes.
5. Once done, allow to release pressure naturally. Remove lid.
6. Serve and enjoy.

NUTRITION: Calories 396 Fat 18 g Carbohydrates 3.5 g Sugar 1.7 g Protein 52.4 g Cholesterol 152 mg

326. Thyme Ginger Garlic Beef

Preparation Time: 10 minutes

Cooking Time: 45 minutes

Servings: 2

INGREDIENTS

- 1 lb beef roast
- 2 whole cloves
- 1/2 tsp ginger, grated
- 1/2 cup beef stock
- 1/2 tsp garlic powder
- 1/2 tsp thyme
- 1/4 tsp pepper
- 1/4 tsp salt

DIRECTIONS

1. Mix together ginger, cloves, thyme, garlic powder, pepper, and salt and rub over beef.
2. Place meat into the instant pot. Pour stock around the meat.

3. Seal pot with lid and cook on high for 45 minutes.
4. Once done, release pressure using quick release. Remove lid.
5. Shred meat using a fork and serve.

NUTRITION: Calories 452 Fat 15.7 g Carbohydrates 5.2 g Sugar 0.4 g Protein 70.1 g Cholesterol 203 mg

327. Beef Shawarma

Preparation Time: 10 minutes

Cooking Time: 10 minutes

Servings: 2

INGREDIENTS

- 1/2 lb ground beef
- 1/4 tsp cinnamon
- 1/2 tsp dried oregano
- 1 cup cabbage, cut into strips
- 1/2 cup bell pepper, sliced
- 1/4 tsp ground coriander
- 1/4 tsp cumin
- 1/4 tsp cayenne pepper
- 1/4 tsp ground allspice
- 1/2 cup onion, chopped
- 1/2 tsp salt

DIRECTIONS

1. Set instant pot on sauté mode.
2. Add meat to the pot and sauté until brown.
3. Add remaining ingredients and stir well.
4. Seal pot with lid and cook on high for 5 minutes.
5. Once done, release pressure using quick release. Remove lid.

6. Stir and serve.

NUTRITION: Calories 245 Fat 7.4 g Carbohydrates 7.9 g Sugar 3.9 g Protein 35.6 g Cholesterol 101 mg

328. Beef Curry

Preparation Time: 10 minutes

Cooking Time: 30 minutes

Servings: 2

INGREDIENTS

- 1/2 lb beef stew meat, cubed
- 1 bell peppers, sliced
- 1 cup beef stock
- 1 tbsp fresh ginger, grated
- 1/2 tsp ground cumin
- 1 tsp ground coriander
- 1/2 tsp cayenne pepper
- 1/2 cup sun-roasted tomatoes, diced
- 2 tbsp olive oil
- 1 tsp garlic, crushed
- 1 green chili peppers, chopped

DIRECTIONS

1. Add all ingredients into the instant pot and stir well.
2. Seal pot with lid and cook on high for 30 minutes.
3. Once done, allow to release pressure naturally. Remove lid.
4. Serve and enjoy.

NUTRITION: Calories 391 Fat 21.9 g Carbohydrates 11.6 g Sugar 5.8 g Protein 37.4 g Cholesterol 101 mg

EGGS RECIPES

329. Breakfast Egg on Avocado

Servings: 6

Cooking Time: 15 minutes

INGREDIENTS

- 1 tsp garlic powder
- 1/2 tsp sea salt
- 1/4 cup Parmesan cheese (grated or shredded)
- 1/4 tsp black pepper
- 3 medium avocados (cut in half, pitted, skin on)
- 6 medium eggs

DIRECTIONS

1. Prepare muffin tins and preheat the oven to 350oF.
2. To ensure that the egg would fit inside the cavity of the avocado, lightly scrape off 1/3 of the meat.
3. Place avocado on muffin tin to ensure that it faces with the top up.
4. Evenly season each avocado with pepper, salt, and garlic powder.
5. Add one egg on each avocado cavity and garnish tops with cheese.
6. Pop in the oven and bake until the egg white is set, about 15 minutes.
7. Serve and enjoy.

NUTRITION: Calories: 252; Protein: 14.0g; Carbs: 4.0g; Fat: 20.0g

330. Breakfast Egg-Artichoke Casserole

Servings: 8

Cooking Time: 35 minutes

INGREDIENTS

- 16 large eggs
- 14 ounce can artichoke hearts, drained
- 10-ounce box frozen chopped spinach, thawed and drained well
- 1 cup shredded white cheddar
- 1 garlic clove, minced
- 1 teaspoon salt
- 1/2 cup parmesan cheese
- 1/2 cup ricotta cheese
- 1/2 teaspoon dried thyme
- 1/2 teaspoon crushed red pepper
- 1/4 cup milk
- 1/4 cup shaved onion

DIRECTIONS

1. Lightly grease a 9x13-inch baking dish with cooking spray and preheat the oven to 350oF.
2. In a large mixing bowl, add eggs and milk. Mix thoroughly.
3. With a paper towel, squeeze out the excess moisture from the spinach leaves and add to the bowl of eggs.
4. Into small pieces, break the artichoke hearts and separate the leaves. Add to the bowl of eggs.
5. Except for the ricotta cheese, add remaining ingredients in the bowl of eggs and mix thoroughly.

6. Pour egg mixture into the prepared dish.
7. Evenly add dollops of ricotta cheese on top of the eggs and then pop in the oven.
8. Bake until eggs are set and doesn't jiggle when shook, about 35 minutes.
9. Remove from the oven and evenly divide into suggested servings. Enjoy.

NUTRITION: Calories: 302; Protein: 22.6g; Carbs: 10.8g; Fat: 18.7g

331. <u>**Brekky Egg-Potato Hash**</u>

Servings: 2,

Cooking Time: 25 minutes

INGREDIENTS

- 1 zucchini, diced
- 1/2 cup chicken broth
- ½ pound cooked chicken
- 1 tablespoon olive oil
- 4 ounces shrimp
- salt and ground black pepper to taste
- 1 large sweet potato, diced
- 2 eggs
- 1/4 teaspoon cayenne pepper
- 2 teaspoons garlic powder
- 1 cup fresh spinach (optional)

DIRECTIONS

1. In a skillet, add the olive oil.
2. Fry the shrimp, cooked chicken and sweet potato for 2 minutes.
3. Add the cayenne pepper, garlic powder and salt and toss for 4 minutes.
4. Add the zucchini and toss for another 3 minutes.

5. Whisk the eggs in a bowl and add to the skillet.
6. Season using salt and pepper. Cover with the lid.
7. Cook for 1 minute and add the chicken broth.
8. Cover and cook for another 8 minutes on high heat.
9. Add the spinach and toss for 2 more minutes.
10. Serve immediately.

NUTRITION: Calories: 190; Protein: 11.7g; Carbs: 2.9g; Fat: 12.3g

332. <u>**Cooked Beef Mushroom Egg**</u>

Servings: 2,

Cooking Time: 15 minutes

INGREDIENTS

- ¼ cup cooked beef, diced
- 6 eggs
- 4 mushrooms, diced
- Salt and pepper to taste
- 12 ounces spinach
- 2 onions, chopped
- A dash of onion powder
- ¼ green bell pepper, chopped
- A dash of garlic powder

DIRECTIONS

1. In a skillet, toss the beef for 3 minutes or until crispy.
2. Take off the heat and add to a plate.
3. Add the onion, bell pepper, and mushroom in the skillet.
4. Add the rest of the ingredients.
5. Toss for about 4 minutes.
6. Return the beef to the skillet and toss for another minute.

7. Serve hot.

NUTRITION:Calories: 213; Protein: 14.5g; Carbs: 3.4g; Fat: 15.7g

333. Curried Veggies and Poached Eggs

Servings: 4,

Cooking Time: 45 minutes

INGREDIENTS

- 4 large eggs
- ½ tsp white vinegar
- 1/8 tsp crushed red pepper – optional
- 1 cup water
- 1 14-oz can chickpeas, drained
- 2 medium zucchinis, diced
- ½ lb sliced button mushrooms
- 1 tbsp yellow curry powder
- 2 cloves garlic, minced
- 1 large onion, chopped
- 2 tsps extra virgin olive oil

DIRECTIONS

1. On medium high fire, place a large saucepan and heat oil.
2. Sauté onions until tender around four to five minutes.
3. Add garlic and continue sautéing for another half minute.
4. Add curry powder, stir and cook until fragrant around one to two minutes.
5. Add mushrooms, mix, cover and cook for 5 to 8 minutes or until mushrooms are tender and have released their liquid.
6. Add red pepper if using, water, chickpeas and zucchini. Mix well to combine and bring to a boil.

7. Once boiling, reduce fire to a simmer, cover and cook until zucchini is tender around 15 to 20 minutes of simmering.
8. Meanwhile, in a small pot filled with 3-inches deep of water, bring to a boil on high fire.
9. Once boiling, reduce fire to a simmer and add vinegar.
10. Slowly add one egg, slipping it gently into the water. Allow to simmer until egg is cooked, around 3 to 5 minutes.
11. Remove egg with a slotted spoon and transfer to a plate, one plate one egg.
12. Repeat the process with remaining eggs.
13. Once the veggies are done cooking, divide evenly into 4 servings and place one serving per plate of egg.
14. Serve and enjoy.

NUTRITION:Calories: 215; Protein: 13.8g; Carbs: 20.6g; Fat: 9.4g

334. Dill and Tomato Frittata

Servings: 6,

Cooking Time: 35 minutes

INGREDIENTS

- pepper and salt to taste
- 1 tsp red pepper flakes
- 2 garlic cloves, minced
- ½ cup crumbled goat cheese – optional
- 2 tbsp fresh chives, chopped
- 2 tbsp fresh dill, chopped
- 4 tomatoes, diced
- 8 eggs, whisked
- 1 tsp coconut oil

DIRECTIONS

1. Grease a 9-inch round baking pan and preheat oven to 325oF.
2. In a large bowl, mix well all ingredients and pour into prepped pan.
3. Pop into the oven and bake until middle is cooked through around 30-35 minutes.
4. Remove from oven and garnish with more chives and dill.

NUTRITION: Calories: ; Protein: ; g; Fat:

335. Dill, Havarti & Asparagus Frittata

Servings: 4,

Cooking Time: 20 minutes

INGREDIENTS

- 1 tsp dried dill weed or 2 tsp minced fresh dill
- 4-oz Havarti cheese cut into small cubes
- 6 eggs, beaten well
- Pepper and salt to taste
- 1 stalk green onions sliced for garnish
- 3 tsp. olive oil
- 2/3 cup diced cherry tomatoes
- 6-8 oz fresh asparagus, ends trimmed and cut into 1 ½-inch lengths

DIRECTIONS

1. On medium-high the fire, place a large cast-iron pan and add oil. Once oil is hot, stir-fry asparagus for 4 minutes.
2. Add dill weed and tomatoes. Cook for two minutes.
3. Meanwhile, season eggs with pepper and salt. Beat well.
4. Pour eggs over the tomatoes.
5. Evenly spread cheese on top.
6. Preheat broiler.
7. Lower the fire to low, cover pan, and let it cook for 10 minutes until the cheese on top has melted.
8. Turn off the fire and transfer pan in the oven and broil for 2 minutes or until tops are browned.
9. Remove from the oven, sprinkle sliced green onions, serve, and enjoy.

NUTRITION: Calories: 244; Protein: 16.0g; Carbs: 3.7g; Fat: 18.3g

336. Egg and Ham Breakfast Cup

Servings: 12,

Cooking Time: 12 minutes

INGREDIENTS

- 2 green onion bunch, chopped
- 12 eggs
- 6 thick pieces nitrate free ham

DIRECTIONS

1. Grease a 12-muffin tin and preheat oven to 400oF.
2. Add 2 hams per muffin compartment, press down to form a cup and add egg in middle. Repeat process to remaining muffin compartments.
3. Pop in the oven and bake until eggs are cooked to desired doneness, around 10 to 12 minutes.
4. To serve, garnish with chopped green onions.

NUTRITION: Calories: 92; Protein: 7.3g; Carbs: 0.8g; Fat: 6.4g

The super Easy Mediterranean Diet Cookbook for Beginners

337. Egg Muffin Sandwich

Servings: 2,

Cooking Time: 10 minutes

Muffin INGREDIENTS

- 1 large egg, free-range or organic
- 1/4 cup almond flour (25 g / 0.9 oz)
- 1/4 cup flax meal (38 g / 1.3 oz)
- 1/4 cup grated cheddar cheese (28 g / 1 oz)
- 1/4 tsp baking soda
- 2 tbsp heavy whipping cream or coconut milk
- 2 tbsp water
- pinch salt

Filing INGREDIENTS

- 1 tbsp butter or 2 tbsp cream cheese for spreading
- 1 tbsp ghee
- 1 tsp Dijon mustard
- 2 large eggs, free-range or organic
- 2 slices cheddar cheese or other hard type cheese (56 g / 2 oz)
- Optional: 1 cup greens (lettuce, kale, chard, spinach, watercress, etc.)
- salt and pepper to taste

DIRECTIONS

- Make the Muffin: In a small mixing bowl, mix well almond flour, flax meal, baking soda, and salt. Stir in water, cream, and eggs. Mix thoroughly.
- Fold in cheese and evenly divide in two single-serve ramekins.
- Pop in the microwave and cook for 75 seconds.

- Make the filing: on medium the fire, place a small nonstick pan, heat ghee and cook the eggs to the desired doneness. Season with pepper and salt.
- To make the muffin sandwiches, slice the muffins in half. Spread cream cheese on one side and mustard on the other side.
- Add egg and greens. Top with the other half of sliced muffin.
- Serve and enjoy.

NUTRITION:Calories: 639; Protein: 26.5g; Carbs: 10.4g; Fat: 54.6g

338. Eggs Benedict and Artichoke Hearts

Servings: 2,

Cooking Time: 30 minutes

INGREDIENTS

- Salt and pepper to taste
- ¾ cup balsamic vinegar
- 4 artichoke hearts
- ¼ cup bacon, cooked
- 1 egg white
- 8 eggs
- 1 tablespoon lemon juice
- ¾ cup melted ghee or butter

DIRECTIONS

1. Line a baking sheet with parchment paper or foil.
2. Preheat the oven to 3750F.
3. Deconstruct the artichokes and remove the hearts. Place the hearts in balsamic vinegar for 20 minutes. Set aside.

4. Prepare the hollandaise sauce by using four (eggs and separate the yolk from the white. Reserve the egg white for the artichoke hearts. Add the yolks and lemon juice and cook in a double boiler while stirring constantly to create a silky texture of the sauce. Add the oil and season with salt and pepper. Set aside.

5. Remove the artichoke hearts from the balsamic vinegar marinade and place on the cookie sheet. Brush the artichokes with the egg white and cook in the oven for 20 minutes.

6. Poach the remaining four (eggs. Turn up the heat and let the water boil. Crack the eggs one at a time and cook for a minute before removing the egg.

7. Assemble by layering the artichokes, bacon and poached eggs.

8. Pour over the hollandaise sauce.

9. Serve with toasted bread.

NUTRITION: Calories: 640; Protein: 28.3g; Carbs: 36.0g; Fat: 42.5g

339. <u>Eggs over Kale Hash</u>

Servings: 4,

Cooking Time: 20 minutes

INGREDIENTS

- 4 large eggs
- 1 bunch chopped kale
- Dash of ground nutmeg
- 2 sweet potatoes, cubed
- 1 14.5-ounce can of chicken broth

DIRECTIONS

1. In a large non-stick skillet, bring the chicken broth to a simmer. Add the sweet potatoes and season slightly with salt and pepper. Add a dash of nutmeg to improve the flavor.

2. Cook until the sweet potatoes become soft, around 10 minutes. Add kale and season with salt and pepper. Continue cooking for four minutes or until kale has wilted. Set aside.

3. Using the same skillet, heat 1 tablespoon of olive oil over medium high heat.

4. Cook the eggs sunny side up until the whites become opaque and the yolks have set. Top the kale hash with the eggs. Serve immediately.

NUTRITION: Calories: 158; Protein: 9.8g; Carbs 18.5g; Fat: 5.6g

340. <u>Eggs with Dill, Pepper, and Salmon</u>

Servings: 6,

Cooking Time: 15 minutes

INGREDIENTS

- pepper and salt to taste
- 1 tsp red pepper flakes
- 2 garlic cloves, minced
- ½ cup crumbled goat cheese
- 2 tbsp fresh chives, chopped
- 2 tbsp fresh dill, chopped
- 4 tomatoes, diced
- 8 eggs, whisked
- 1 tsp coconut oil

DIRECTIONS

1. In a big bowl whisk the eggs. Mix in pepper, salt, red pepper flakes, garlic, dill and salmon.

2. On low fire, place a nonstick fry pan and lightly grease with oil.
3. Pour egg mixture and whisk around until cooked through to make scrambled eggs.
4. Serve and enjoy topped with goat cheese.

NUTRITION:Calories: 141; Protein: 10.3g; Carbs: 6.7g; Fat: 8.5g

341. Fig and Walnut Skillet Frittata

Servings: 4,

Cooking Time: 15 minutes

INGREDIENTS

- 1 cup figs, halved
- 4 eggs, beaten
- 1 teaspoon cinnamon
- A pinch of salt
- 2 tablespoons almond flour
- 2 tablespoons coconut flour
- 1 cup walnut, chopped
- 2 tablespoons coconut oil
- 1 teaspoon cardamom
- 6 tablespoons raw honey

DIRECTIONS

1. In a mixing bowl, beat the eggs.
2. Add the coconut flour, almond flour, cardamom, honey, salt and cinnamon.
3. Mix well. Heat the coconut oil in a skillet over medium heat.
4. Add the egg mixture gently.
5. Add the walnuts and figs on top.
6. Cover and cook on medium low heat for about 10 minutes.
7. Serve hot with more honey on top.

NUTRITION:Calories: 221; Protein: 12.7g; Carbs: 5.9g; Fat: 16.3g

342. Frittata with Dill and Tomatoes

Servings: 4,

Cooking Time: 35 minutes

INGREDIENTS

- pepper and salt to taste
- 1 tsp red pepper flakes
- 2 garlic cloves, minced
- ½ cup crumbled goat cheese – optional
- 2 tbsp fresh chives, chopped
- 2 tbsp fresh dill, chopped
- 4 tomatoes, diced
- 8 eggs, whisked
- 1 tsp coconut oil

DIRECTIONS

1. Grease a 9-inch round baking pan and preheat oven to 325oF.
2. In a large bowl, mix well all ingredients and pour into prepped pan.
3. Pop into the oven and bake until middle is cooked through around 30-35 minutes.
4. Remove from oven and garnish with more chives and dill.

NUTRITION:Calories: 309; Protein: 19.8g; Carbs: 8.0g; Fat: 22.0g

343. Italian Scrambled Eggs

Servings: 1,

Cooking Time: 7 minutes

INGREDIENTS

- 1 teaspoon balsamic vinegar
- 2 large eggs
- ¼ teaspoon rosemary, minced
- ½ cup cherry tomatoes
- 1 ½ cup kale, chopped
- ½ teaspoon olive oil

DIRECTIONS

1. Melt the olive oil in a skillet over medium high heat.
2. Sauté the kale and add rosemary and salt to taste. Add three tablespoons of water to prevent the kale from burning at the bottom of the pan. Cook for three to four minutes.
3. Add the tomatoes and stir.
4. Push the vegetables on one side of the skillet and add the eggs. Season with salt and pepper to taste.
5. Scramble the eggs then fold in the tomatoes and kales.

NUTRITION: Calories: 230; Protein: 16.4g; Carbs: 15.0g; Fat: 12.4g

344. Kale and Red Pepper Frittata

Servings: 4,

Cooking Time: 23 minutes

INGREDIENTS

- Salt and pepper to taste
- ½ cup almond milk
- 8 large eggs
- 2 cups kale, rinsed and chopped
- 3 slices of crispy bacon, chopped
- 1/3 cup onion, chopped
- ½ cup red pepper, chopped
- 1 tablespoon coconut oil

DIRECTIONS

1. Preheat the oven to 3500F.
2. In a medium bowl, combine the eggs and almond milk. Season with salt and pepper. Set aside.
3. In a skillet, heat the coconut oil over medium flame and sauté the onions and red pepper for three minutes or until the onion is translucent. Add in the kale and cook for 5 minutes more.
4. Add the eggs into the mixture along with the bacon and cook for four minutes or until the edges start to set.
5. Continue cooking the frittata in the oven for 15 minutes.

NUTRITION: Calories: 242; Protein: 16.5g; Carbs: 7.0g; Fat: 16.45g

345. Lettuce Stuffed with Eggs 'n Crab Meat

Servings: 8,

Cooking Time: 10 minutes

INGREDIENTS

- 24 butter lettuce leaves
- 1 tsp dry mustard
- ¼ cup finely chopped celery
- 1 cup lump crabmeat, around 5 ounces
- 3 tbsp plain Greek yogurt
- 2 tbsp extra virgin olive oil
- ¼ tsp ground pepper
- 8 large eggs
- ½ tsp salt, divided
- 1 tbsp fresh lemon juice, divided
- 2 cups thinly sliced radishes

DIRECTIONS

1. In a medium bowl, mix ¼ tsp salt, 2 tsps. juice and radishes. Cover and chill for half an hour.
2. On medium saucepan, place eggs and cover with water over an inch above the eggs. Bring the pan of water to a boil. Once boiling, reduce fire to a simmer and cook for ten minutes.
3. Turn off fire, discard hot water and place eggs in an ice water bath to cool completely.
4. Peel eggshells and slice eggs in half lengthwise and remove the yolks.
5. With a sieve on top of a bowl, place yolks and press through a sieve. Set aside a tablespoon of yolk.
6. On remaining bowl of yolks add pepper, ¼ tsp salt and 1 tsp juice. Mix well and as you are stirring, slowly add oil until well incorporated. Add yogurt, stir well to mix.
7. Add mustard, celery and crabmeat. Gently mix to combine. If needed, taste and adjust seasoning of the filling.
8. On a serving platter, arrange 3 lettuce in a fan for two egg slices. To make the egg whites sit flat, you can slice a bit of the bottom to make it flat. Evenly divide crab filling into egg white holes.
9. Then evenly divide into eight servings the radish salad and add on the side of the eggs, on top of the lettuce leaves. Serve and enjoy.

NUTRITION: Calories: 121; Protein: 10.0g; Carbs: 1.6g; Fat: 8.3g

346. <u>Mixed Greens and Ricotta Frittata</u>

Servings: 8,

Cooking Time: 35 minutes

INGREDIENTS

- 1 tbsp pine nuts
- 1 clove garlic, chopped
- ¼ cup fresh mint leaves
- ¾ cup fresh parsley leaves
- 1 cup fresh basil leaves
- 8-oz part-skim ricotta
- 1 tbsp red-wine vinegar
- ½ + 1/8 tsp freshly ground black pepper, divided
- ½ tsp salt, divided
- 10 large eggs
- 1 lb chopped mixed greens
- Pinch of red pepper flakes
- 1 medium red onion, finely diced
- 1/3 cup + 2 tbsp olive oil, divided

DIRECTIONS

1. Preheat oven to 350oF.
2. On medium high fire, place a nonstick skillet and heat 1 tbsp oil. Sauté onions until soft and translucent, around 4 minutes. Add half of greens and pepper flakes and sauté until tender and crisp, around 5 minutes. Remove cooked greens and place in colander. Add remaining uncooked greens in skillet and sauté until tender and crisp, when done add to colander. Allow cooked veggies to cool enough to handle, then squeeze dry and place in a bowl.
3. Whisk well ¼ tsp pepper, ¼ tsp salt, Parmesan and eggs in a large bowl.

4. In bowl of cooked vegetables, add 1/8 tsp pepper, ricotta and vinegar. Mix thoroughly. Then pour into bowl of eggs and mix well.

5. On medium fire, place same skillet used previously and heat 1 tbsp oil. Pour egg mixture and cook for 8 minutes or until sides are set. Turn off fire, place skillet inside oven and bake for 15 minutes or until middle of frittata is set.

6. Meanwhile, make the pesto by processing pine nuts, garlic, mint, parsley and basil in a food processor until coarsely chopped. Add 1/3 cup oil and continue processing. Season with remaining pepper and salt. Process once again until thoroughly mixed.

7. To serve, slice the frittata in 8 equal wedges and serve with a dollop of pesto.

NUTRITION: Calories: 280; Protein: 14g; Carbs: 8g; Fat: 21.3g

347. <u>Mushroom Tomato Frittata</u>

Servings: 8,

Cooking Time: 8 minutes

INGREDIENTS

- ¼ cup mushroom, sliced
- 10 eggs
- 1 cup cherry tomatoes
- Salt
- Pepper
- 1 teaspoon olive oil

DIRECTIONS

1. Whisk the eggs in a bowl.
2. Add the eggs in a skillet.

3. Add the mushroom, cherry tomatoes and season using salt and pepper.
4. Cover with lid and cook for about 5 to 8 minutes on low heat.

NUTRITION: Calories: 190; Protein: 11.7g; Carbs: 2.9g; Fat: 12.3g

348. <u>Mushroom, Spinach and Turmeric Frittata</u>

Servings: 6,

Cooking Time: 35 minutes

INGREDIENTS

- ½ tsp pepper
- ½ tsp salt
- 1 tsp turmeric
- 5-oz firm tofu
- 4 large eggs
- 6 large egg whites
- ¼ cup water
- 1 lb fresh spinach
- 6 cloves freshly chopped garlic
- 1 large onion, chopped
- 1 lb button mushrooms, sliced

DIRECTIONS

1. Grease a 10-inch nonstick and oven proof skillet and preheat oven to 350oF.
2. Place skillet on medium high fire and add mushrooms. Cook until golden brown.
3. Add onions, cook for 3 minutes or until onions are tender.
4. Add garlic, sauté for 30 seconds.
5. Add water and spinach, cook while covered until spinach is wilted, around 2 minutes.

6. Remove lid and continue cooking until water is fully evaporated.
7. In a blender, puree pepper, salt, turmeric, tofu, eggs and egg whites until smooth. Pour into skillet once liquid is fully evaporated.
8. Pop skillet into oven and bake until the center is set around 25-30 minutes.
9. Remove skillet from oven and let it stand for ten minutes before inverting and transferring to a serving plate.
10. Cut into 6 equal wedges, serve and enjoy.

NUTRITION:Calories: 166; Protein: 15.9g; Carbs: 12.2g; Fat: 6.0g

349. Paleo Almond Banana Pancakes

Servings: 3,

Cooking Time: 10 minutes

INGREDIENTS

- ¼ cup almond flour
- ½ teaspoon ground cinnamon
- 3 eggs
- 1 banana, mashed
- 1 tablespoon almond butter
- 1 teaspoon vanilla extract
- 1 teaspoon olive oil
- Sliced banana to serve

DIRECTIONS

1. Whisk the eggs in a mixing bowl until they become fluffy.
2. In another bowl mash the banana using a fork and add to the egg mixture.
3. Add the vanilla, almond butter, cinnamon and almond flour.

4. Mix into a smooth batter.
5. Heat the olive oil in a skillet.
6. Add one spoonful of the batter and fry them from both sides.
7. Keep doing these steps until you are done with all the batter.
8. Add some sliced banana on top before serving.

NUTRITION:Calories: 306; Protein: 14.4g; Carbs: 3.6g; Fat: 26.0g

350. Parmesan and Poached Eggs on Asparagus

Servings: 4,

Cooking Time: 15 minutes

INGREDIENTS

- 4 tbsp coarsely grated fresh Parmesan cheese, divided
- Freshly ground black pepper, to taste
- 2 tsps finely chopped fresh parsley
- 2 tbsp fresh lemon juice
- 1 tbsp unsalted butter
- 1 garlic clove, chopped
- 1 tbsp extra virgin olive oil
- 2 bunches asparagus spears, trimmed around 40
- 1 tsp salt, divided
- 1 tsp white vinegar
- 8 large eggs

DIRECTIONS

1. Break eggs and place in one paper cup per egg. On medium high fire, place a low sided pan filled 3/4 with water. Add ½ tsp salt and vinegar into water. Set aside.
2. On medium high fire bring another pot of water to boil. Once boiling, lower

fire to a simmer and blanch asparagus until tender and crisp, around 3-4 minutes. With tongs transfer asparagus to a serving platter and set aside.

3. On medium fire, place a medium saucepan and heat olive oil. Once hot, for a minute sauté garlic and turn off fire. Add butter right away and swirl around pan to melt. Add remaining pepper, salt, parsley and lemon juice and mix thoroughly. Add asparagus and toss to combine well with garlic butter sauce. Transfer to serving platter along with sauce.

4. In boiling pan of water, poach the eggs by pouring eggs into the water slowly and cook for two minutes per egg. With a slotted spoon, remove egg, to remove excess water, tap slotted spoon several times on kitchen towel and place on top of asparagus.

5. To serve, top eggs with parmesan cheese and divide the asparagus into two and 2 eggs per plate. Serve and enjoy.

NUTRITION: Calories: 256; Protein: 18g; Carbs: 8g; Fat: 16.9g

351. Scrambled Eggs with Feta 'n Mushrooms

Servings: 1

Cooking Time: 6 minutes

INGREDIENTS

- Pepper to taste
- 2 tbsp feta cheese
- 1 whole egg
- 2 egg whites
- 1 cup fresh spinach, chopped
- ½ cup fresh mushrooms, sliced
- Cooking spray

DIRECTIONS

1. On medium high fire, place a nonstick fry pan and grease with cooking spray.
2. Once hot, add spinach and mushrooms.
3. Sauté until spinach is wilted, around 2-3 minutes.
4. Meanwhile, in a bowl whisk well egg, egg whites, and cheese. Season with pepper.
5. Pour egg mixture into pan and scramble until eggs are cooked through, around 3-4 minutes.
6. Serve and enjoy with a piece of toast or brown rice.

NUTRITION: Calories: 211; Protein: 18.6g; Carbs: 7.4g; Fat: 11.9g

352. Scrambled eggs with Smoked Salmon

Servings: 1,

Cooking Time: 8 minutes

INGREDIENTS

- 1 tbsp coconut oil
- Pepper and salt to taste
- 1/8 tsp red pepper flakes
- 1/8 tsp garlic powder
- 1 tbsp fresh dill, chopped finely
- 4 oz smoked salmon, torn apart
- 2 whole eggs + 1 egg yolk, whisked

DIRECTIONS

1. In a big bowl whisk the eggs. Mix in pepper, salt, red pepper flakes, garlic, dill and salmon.
2. On low fire, place a nonstick fry pan and lightly grease with oil.
3. Pour egg mixture and whisk around until cooked through to make scrambled eggs, around 8 minutes on medium fire.
4. Serve and enjoy.

NUTRITION: Calories: 366; Protein: 32.0; Carbs: 1.0g; Fat: 26.0g

353. Spiced Breakfast Casserole

Servings: 6,

Cooking Time: 35 minutes

INGREDIENTS

- 1 tablespoon nutrition al yeast
- ¼ cup water
- 6 large eggs
- 1 teaspoon coriander
- 1 teaspoon cumin
- 8 kale leaves, stems removed and torn into small pieces
- 2 sausages, cooked and chopped
- 1 large sweet potato, peeled and chopped

DIRECTIONS

1. Preheat the oven to 375oF.
2. Grease an 8" x 8" baking pan with olive oil and set aside.
3. Place sweet potatoes in a microwavable bowl and add ¼ cup water. Cook the chopped sweet potatoes in the microwave for three to

five minutes. Drain the excess water then set aside.
4. Fry in a skillet heated over medium flame the sausage and cook until brown. Mix in the kale and cook until wilted.
5. Add the coriander, cumin and cooked sweet potatoes.
6. In another bowl, mix together the eggs, water and nutritional yeast. Add the vegetable and meat mixture into the bowl and mix completely.
7. Place the mixture in the baking dish and make sure that the mixture is evenly distributed within the pan.
8. Bake for 20 minutes or until the eggs are done.
9. Slice into squares.

NUTRITION: Calories: 137; Protein: 10.1g; Carbs: 10.0g; Fat: 6.6g

354. Spinach, Mushroom and Sausage Frittata

Servings: 4,

Cooking Time: 30 minutes

INGREDIENTS

- Salt and pepper to taste
- 10 eggs
- ½ small onion, chopped
- 1 cup mushroom, sliced
- 1 cup fresh spinach, chopped
- ½ pound sausage, ground
- 2 tablespoon coconut oil

DIRECTIONS

1. Preheat the oven to 3500F.
2. Heat a skillet over medium high flame and add the coconut oil.

3. Sauté the onions until softened. Add in the sausage and cook for two minutes

4. Add in the spinach and mushroom. Stir constantly until the spinach has wilted.

5. Turn off the stove and distribute the vegetable mixture evenly.

6. Pour in the beaten eggs and transfer to the oven.

7. Cook for twenty minutes or until the eggs are completely cooked through.

NUTRITION: Calories: 383; Protein: 24.9g; Carbs: 8.6g; Fat: 27.6g

355. <u>Tomato-Bacon Quiche</u>

Servings: 6,

Cooking Time: 47 minutes

Topping INGREDIENTS

- 2 small medium sized tomatoes, sliced

Quiche INGREDIENTS

- ¼ tsp black pepper
- ¼ tsp salt
- ¼ tsp ground mustard
- ½ cup fresh spinach, chopped
- 2/4 cups cauliflower, ground into rice
- 5 slices nitrate free bacon, cooked and chopped
- 3 tbsp unsweetened plain almond milk
- ½ cup organic white eggs
- 5 eggs, beaten
- Zucchini Hash Crust:
- 1/8 tsp sea salt
- 1 tbsp butter
- 1 tsp flax meal
- 1 ½ tbsp coconut flour
- 1 egg, beaten

- 2 small to medium sized organic zucchini, grated

DIRECTIONS

1. Grease a pie dish and preheat oven to 400oF.

2. Grate zucchini, drain and squeeze dry.

3. In a bowl, add dry zucchini and remaining crust ingredients and mix well.

4. Place in bottom of pie plate and press down as if making a pie crust. Pop in the oven and bake for 9 minutes.

5. Meanwhile in a large mixing bowl, whisk well black pepper, salt, mustard, almond milk, egg whites, and egg.

6. Add bacon, spinach, and cauliflower rice. Mix well. Pour into baked zucchini crust, top with tomato slices.

7. Pop back in the oven and bake for 28 minutes. If at 20 minutes baking time top is browning too much, cover with parchment paper for remainder of cooking time.

8. Once done cooking, remove from oven, let it stand for at least ten minutes.

9. Slice into equal triangles, serve and enjoy.

NUTRITION: Calories: 154; Protein: 11.6g; Carbs: 3.4g; Fat: 10.3g

356. <u>Your Standard Quiche</u>

Servings: 6,

Cooking Time: 45 minutes

INGREDIENTS

- 4 oz sliced Portobello mushrooms
- pepper and salt to taste

- ½ tbsp dried basil
- ½ tbsp dried parsley
- 6 eggs, whisked
- ¾ lb pork breakfast sausage

DIRECTIONS

1. Grease a 9-inch round pie plate or baking pan and preheat oven to 350oF.
2. On medium fire, place a nonstick fry pan and cook sausage. Stir fry until cooked as you break them into pieces. Discard excess oil once cooked.
3. In a big bowl, whisk pepper, salt, basil, parsley and eggs. Pour into prepped baking plate.
4. Pop into the oven and bake until middle is firm around 30-35 minutes.
5. Once done, remove from oven; let it stand for 10 minutes before slicing and serving.

NUTRITION: Calories: 283; Protein: 15.0g; Carbs: 3.2g; Fat: 23.3g

357. **Zucchini Tomato Frittata**

Servings: 8,

Cooking Time: 30 minutes

INGREDIENTS

- 3 lbs tomatoes, thinly sliced crosswise
- ¾ cup cheddar cheese, shredded
- ¼ cup milk
- 8 large eggs
- 1 tbsp fresh thyme leaves

- 3 zucchinis, cut into ¼-inch thick rounds
- 1 onion, finely chopped
- 1 tbsp olive oil
- Salt and pepper to taste

DIRECTIONS

1. Preheat the oven to 425 degrees Fahrenheit.
2. Prepare a non-stick skillet and heat it over medium heat.
3. Sauté the zucchini, onion and thyme. Cook and stir often for 8 to 10 minutes. Let the liquid in the pan evaporate and season with salt and pepper to taste. Remove the skillet from heat.
4. In a bowl, whisk the milk, cheese, eggs, salt and pepper together. Pour the egg mixture over the zucchini in the skillet. Lift the zucchini to allow the eggs to coat the pan. Arrange the tomato slices on top.
5. Return to the skillet and heat to medium low fire and cook until the sides are set or golden brown, around 7 minutes.
6. Place the skillet inside the oven and cook for 10 to 15 minutes or until the center of the frittata is cooked through. To check if the egg is cooked through, insert a wooden skewer in the middle and it should come out clean.
7. Remove from the oven and loosen the frittata from the skillet. Serve warm.

NUTRITION: Calories: 175; Protein: 12.0g; Carbs: 13.6g; Fat: 8.1g

VEGETARIAN RECIPES

358. Creamy Carrot Chowder

Servings: 8,

Cooking Time: 40 minutes

INGREDIENTS

- 8 fresh mint sprigs
- ½ cup 2% Greek Style Plain yogurt
- 1 tsp fresh ginger, peeled and grated
- 2 cups chicken broth
- 1 lb. baby carrots, peeled and cut into 2-inch lengths
- 1/3 cup sliced shallots
- 2 tsp sesame oil

DIRECTIONS

1. On medium fire, place a medium heavy bottom pot and heat oil.
2. Sauté shallots until tender around 2 minutes.
3. Add carrots and sauté for another 4 minutes.
4. Pour broth, cover and bring to a boil. Once soup is boiling, slow fire to a simmer and cook carrots until tender around 22 minutes.
5. Add ginger and continue cooking while covered for another eight minutes.
6. Turn off fire and let it cool for 10 minutes.
7. Pour mixture into blender and puree. If needed, puree carrots in batches then return to pot.
8. Heat pureed carrots until heated through around 2 minutes.
9. Turn off fire and evenly pour into 8 serving bowls.
10. Serve and enjoy. Or you can store in the freezer in 8 different lidded containers for a quick soup in the middle of the week.

NUTRITION:Calories: 47; Carbs: 6.5g; Protein: 2.2g; Fat: 1.6g

359. Creamy Corn Soup

Servings: 4,

Cooking Time: 20 minutes

INGREDIENTS

- 4 slices crisp cooked bacon, crumbled
- 2 tbsp cornstarch
- 1/4 cup water
- 2 tsp soy sauce
- 4 cups chicken broth
- 1 (14.75 oz) can cream-style corn
- 2 egg whites
- 1/4 tsp salt
- 1 tbsp sherry
- 1/2 lb. skinless, boneless chicken breast meat, finely chopped

DIRECTIONS

1. Combine chicken with the sherry, egg whites, salt in a bowl. Stir in the cream style corn. Mix well.
2. Boil the soy sauce and chicken broth in a wok. Then stir in the chicken mixture, while continue boiling. Then simmer for about 3 minutes, stir frequently to avoid burning.
3. Mix corn starch and water until well combined. Mix to the simmering broth,

while constantly stirring until it slightly thickens. Cook for about 2 minutes more.

4. Serve topped with the crumbled bacon.

NUTRITION: Calories: 305; Carbs: 28.0g; Protein: 21.1g; Fat: 13.0g

360. Creamy Kale and Mushrooms

Servings: 3,

Cooking Time: 15 minutes

INGREDIENTS

- 3 tablespoons coconut oil
- 3 cloves of garlic, minced
- 1 onion, chopped
- 1 bunch kale, stems removed and leaves chopped
- 5 white button mushrooms, chopped
- 1 cup coconut milk
- Salt and pepper to taste

DIRECTIONS

1. Heat oil in a pot.
2. Sauté the garlic and onion until fragrant for 2 minutes.
3. Stir in mushrooms. Season with pepper and salt. Cook for 8 minutes.
4. Stir in kale and coconut milk. Simmer for 5 minutes.
5. Adjust seasoning to taste.

NUTRITION:Calories: 365; Carbs: 17.9g; Protein: 6g; Fat: 33.5g

361. Crunchy Kale Chips

Servings: 8,

Cooking Time: 2 hours

INGREDIENTS

- 2 tbsp filtered water
- ½ tsp sea salt
- 1 tbsp raw honey
- 2 tbsp nutrition al yeast
- 1 lemon, juiced
- 1 cup sweet potato, grated
- 1 cup fresh cashews, soaked 2 hours
- 2 bunches green curly kale, washed, ribs and stems removed, leaves torn into bite sized pieces

DIRECTIONS

1. Prepare a baking sheet by covering with an unbleached parchment paper. Preheat oven to 150oF.
2. In a large mixing bowl, place kale.
3. In a food processor, process remaining ingredients until smooth. Pour over kale.
4. With your hands, coat kale with marinade.
5. Evenly spread kale onto parchment paper and pop in the oven. Dehydrate for 2 hours and turn leaves after the first hour of baking.
6. Remove from oven; let it cool completely before serving.

NUTRITION:Calories: 209; Carbs: 13.0g; Protein: 7.0g; Fat: 15.9g

362. <u>Delicious and Healthy Roasted Eggplant</u>

Servings: 6,

Cooking Time: 30 minutes

INGREDIENTS

- Pinch of sugar
- ¼ tsp salt
- ¼ tsp cayenne pepper or to taste
- 1 tbsp parsley, flat leaf and chopped finely
- 2 tbsp fresh basil, chopped
- 1 small chili pepper, seeded and minced, optional
- ½ cup red onion, finely chopped
- ½ cup Greek feta cheese, crumbled
- ¼ cup extra virgin olive oil
- 2 tbsp lemon juice
- 1 medium eggplant, around 1 lb.

DIRECTIONS

1. Preheat broiler and position rack 6 inches away from heat source.
2. Pierce the eggplant with a knife or fork. Then with a foil, line a baking pan and place the eggplant and broil. Make sure to turn eggplant every five minutes or until the skin is charred and eggplant is soft which takes around 14 to 18 minutes of broiling. Once done, remove from heat and let cool.
3. In a medium bowl, add lemon. Then cut eggplant in half, lengthwise, and scrape the flesh and place in the bowl with lemon. Add oil and mix until well combined. Then add salt, cayenne, parsley, basil, chili pepper, bell pepper, onion and feta. Toss until well

combined and add sugar to taste if wanted.

NUTRITION: Calories: 97; Carbs: 7.4g; Protein: 2.9g; Fat: 6.7g

363. <u>Delicious Stuffed Squash</u>

Servings: 4 servings,

Cooking Time: 30minutes

INGREDIENTS

- ¼ cup sour cream
- ½ cup shredded cheddar
- 3 tbsp taco sauce
- 1 small tomato, chopped
- ½ small green bell pepper, seeded and chopped
- ½ medium onion, chopped
- 1 tsp cumin
- 1 tsp onion powder
- ¼ tsp cayenne
- 1 ½ tsp chili powder
- 1 can 15-oz black beans, drained and rinsed
- 1 clove garlic, minced
- 1 tbsp olive oil
- 2 medium zucchinis
- 2 medium yellow squash
- Salt and pepper

DIRECTIONS

1. Boil until tender in a large pot of water zucchini and yellow squash, then drain. Lengthwise, slice the squash and trim the ends. Take out the center flesh and chop.
2. On medium high fire, place skillet with oil and sauté garlic until fragrant. Add

onion and tomato and sauté for 8 minutes. Add chopped squash, bell pepper, cumin, onion powder, cayenne, chilli powder and black beans and continue cooking until veggies are tender.

3. Season with pepper and salt to taste. Remove from fire.

4. Spread 1 tsp of taco sauce on each squash shell, fill with half of the cooked filling, top with cheese and garnish with sour cream. Repeat procedure on other half of squash shell. Serve and enjoy.

NUTRITION:Calories: 318; Carbs: 28.0g; Protein: 21.0g; Fat: 16.0g

364. Easy and Healthy Baked Vegetables

Servings: 6,

Cooking Time: 1 hour and 15 minutes

INGREDIENTS

- 2 lbs. Brussels sprouts, trimmed
- 3 lbs. Butternut Squash, peeled, seeded and cut into same size as sprouts
- 1 lb Pork breakfast sausage
- 1 tbsp fat from fried sausage

DIRECTIONS

1. Grease a 9x13 inch baking pan and preheat oven to 350oF.
2. On medium high fire, place a large nonstick saucepan and cook sausage. Break up sausages and cook until browned.
3. In a greased pan mix browned sausage, squash, sprouts, sea salt

and fat. Toss to mix well. Pop into the oven and cook for an hour.

4. Remove from oven and serve warm.

NUTRITION:Calories: 364; Carbs: 41.2g; Protein: 19.0g; Fat: 16.5g

365. Eggplant Bolognese With Zucchini Noodles

Servings: 4,

Cooking Time: 20 minutes

INGREDIENTS

- 6 leaves of fresh basil, chopped
- 1 28-ounce can plum tomatoes
- ½ cup red wine
- 1 tablespoon tomato paste
- 4 sprigs of thyme, chopped
- 2 bay leaves
- 3 cloves garlic, minced
- 1 large yellow onion, chopped
- Salt and pepper to taste
- 2 tablespoon extra-virgin olive oil
- ½ pound ground beef
- 1 ½ pounds eggplant, diced
- 2 cups zucchini noodles

DIRECTIONS

1. Heat the skillet over medium high heat and add oil. Sauté the onion and beef and sprinkle with salt and pepper. Sauté for 10 minutes until the meat is brown. Add in the eggplants, bay leaves, garlic and thyme. Cook for another 15 minutes.
2. Once the eggplant is tender, add the tomato paste and wine. Add the tomatoes and crush using a spoon.

Bring to a boil and reduce the heat to low. Simmer for 10 minutes.

3. In a skillet, add oil and sauté the zucchini noodles for five minutes. Turn off the heat.
4. Pour the tomato sauce over the zucchini noodles and garnish with fresh basil.

NUTRITION: Calories: 320; Carbs: 24.8g; Protein: 19.2g; Fat: 17.0g

366. Feta and Roasted Eggplant Dip

Servings: 12,

Cooking Time: 20 minutes

INGREDIENTS

- ¼ tsp salt
- ¼ tsp cayenne pepper
- 1 tbsp finely chopped flat leaf parsley
- 2 tbsp chopped fresh basil
- 1 small Chile pepper
- 1 small red bell pepper, finely chopped
- ½ cup finely chopped red onion
- ½ cup crumbled Greek nonfat feta cheese
- ¼ cup extra-virgin olive oil
- 2 tbsp lemon juice
- 1 medium eggplant, around 1 lb.

DIRECTIONS

1. Preheat broiler, position rack on topmost part of oven, and line a baking pan with foil.
2. With a fork or knife, poke eggplant, place on prepared baking pan, and broil for 5 minutes per side until skin is charred all around.

3. Once eggplant skin is charred, remove from broiler and allow to cool to handle.
4. Once eggplant is cool enough to handle, slice in half lengthwise, scoop out flesh, and place in a medium bowl.
5. Pour in lemon juice and toss eggplant to coat with lemon juice and prevent it from discoloring.
6. Add oil; continue mixing until oil is absorbed by eggplant.
7. Stir in salt, cayenne pepper, parsley, basil, Chile pepper, bell pepper, onion, and feta.
8. Toss to mix well and serve.

NUTRITION: Calories: 58; Carbs: 3.7g; Protein: 1.2g; Fat: 4.6g

367. Garlic 'n Sour Cream Zucchini Bake

Servings: 3,

Cooking Time: 20 minutes

INGREDIENTS

- 1/4 cup grated Parmesan cheese
- paprika to taste
- 1 tablespoon minced garlic
- 1 large zucchini, cut lengthwise then in half
- 1 cup sour cream
- 1 (8 ounce) package cream cheese, softened

DIRECTIONS

1. Lightly grease a casserole dish with cooking spray.
2. Place zucchini slices in a single layer in dish.

3. In a bowl whisk well, remaining **INGREDIENTS** except for paprika. Spread on top of zucchini slices. Sprinkle paprika.
4. Cover dish with foil.
5. For 10 minutes, cook in preheated 390oF oven.
6. Remove foil and cook for 10 minutes.
7. Serve and enjoy.

NUTRITION: Calories: 385; Carbs: 13.5g; Protein: 11.9g; Fat: 32.4g

368. Garlicky Rosemary Potatoes

Servings: 4,

Cooking Time: 2 minutes

INGREDIENTS

- 1-pound potatoes, peeled and sliced thinly
- 2 garlic cloves
- ½ teaspoon salt
- 1 tablespoon olive oil
- 2 sprigs of rosemary

DIRECTIONS

1. Place a trivet or steamer basket in the Instant Pot and pour in a cup of water.
2. In a baking dish that can fit inside the Instant Pot, combine all ingredients and toss to coat everything.
3. Cover the baking dish with aluminum foil and place on the steamer basket.
4. Close the lid and press the Steam button.
5. Adjust the cooking time to 30 minutes
6. Do quick pressure release.
7. Once cooled, evenly divide into serving size, keep in your preferred container, and refrigerate until ready to eat.

NUTRITION: Calories: 119; Carbs: 20.31g; Protein: 2.39g; Fat: 3.48g

369. Ginger and Spice Carrot Soup

Servings: 6,

Cooking Time: 40 minutes

INGREDIENTS

- ¼ cup Greek yogurt
- 2 tsp fresh lime juice
- 5 cups low-salt chicken broth
- 1 ½ tsp finely grated lime peel
- 4 cups of carrots, peeled, thinly sliced into rounds
- 2 cups chopped onions
- 1 tbsp minced and peeled fresh ginger
- ½ tsp curry powder
- 3 tbsp expeller-pressed sunflower oil
- ½ tsp yellow mustard seeds
- 1 tsp coriander seeds

DIRECTIONS

1. In a food processor, grind mustard seeds and coriander into a powder.
2. On medium high fire, place a large pot and heat oil.
3. Add curry powder and powdered seeds and sauté for a minute.
4. Add ginger, cook for a minute.
5. Add lime peel, carrots and onions. Sauté for 3 minutes or until onions are softened.
6. Season with pepper and salt.

7. Add broth and bring to a boil. Reduce fire to a simmer and simmer uncovered for 30 minutes or until carrots are tender.
8. Cool broth slightly, and puree in batches. Return pureed carrots into pot.
9. Add lime juice, add more pepper and salt to taste.
10. Transfer to a serving bowl, drizzle with yogurt and serve.

NUTRITION: Calories: 129; Carbs: 13.6g; Protein: 2.8g; Fat: 7.7g

370. Ginger-Egg Drop Soup with Zoodle

Servings: 4,

Cooking Time: 15 minutes

INGREDIENTS

- ½ teaspoons red pepper flakes
- 2 cups thinly sliced scallions, divided
- 2 cups, plus 1 tablespoon water, divided
- 2 tablespoons extra virgin olive oil
- 2 tablespoons minced ginger
- 3 tablespoons corn starch
- 4 large eggs, beaten
- 4 medium to large zucchini, spiralized into noodles
- 5 cups shiitake mushrooms, sliced
- 5 tablespoons low-sodium tamari sauce or soy sauce
- 8 cups vegetable broth, divided
- Salt & pepper to taste

DIRECTIONS

1. On medium-high the fire, place a large pot and add oil.
2. Once oil is hot, stir in ginger and sauté for two minutes.
3. Stir in a tablespoon of water and shiitake mushrooms. Cook for 5 minutes or until mushrooms start to give off liquid.
4. Stir in 1 ½ cups scallions, tamari sauce, red pepper flakes, remaining water, and 7 cups of the vegetable broth. Mix well and bring to a boil.
5. Meanwhile, in a small bowl whisk well cornstarch and remaining cup of vegetable broth and set aside.
6. Once pot is boiling, slowly pour in eggs while stirring pot continuously. Mix well.
7. Add the cornstarch slurry in pot and mix well. Continue mixing every now and then until thickened, about 5 minutes.
8. Taste and adjust seasoning with pepper and salt.
9. Stir in zoodles and cook until heated through, about 2 minutes.
10. Serve with a sprinkle of remaining scallions and enjoy.

NUTRITION: Calories: 238; Protein: 10.6g; Carbs: 34.3g; Sugar: 12.8g; Fat: 8.6g

371. Ginger Vegetable Stir Fry

Servings: 4,

Cooking Time: 5 minutes

INGREDIENTS

- 1 tablespoon oil
- 3 cloves of garlic, minced
- 1 onion, chopped
- 1 thumb-size ginger, sliced

- 1 tablespoon water
- 1 large carrots, peeled and julienned
- 1 large green bell pepper, seeded and julienned
- 1 large yellow bell pepper, seeded and julienned
- 1 large red bell pepper, seeded and julienned
- 1 zucchini, julienned
- Salt and pepper to taste

DIRECTIONS

1. Heat oil in a skillet over medium flame and sauté the garlic, onion, and ginger until fragrant.
2. Stir in the rest of the ingredients and adjust the flame to high.
3. Keep on stirring for at least 5 minutes until vegetables are half-cooked.
4. Place in individual containers.
5. Put a label and store in the fridge.
6. Allow to thaw at room temperature before heating in the microwave oven.

NUTRITION: Calories: 102; Carbs: 13.6g; Protein:0 g; Fat: 2g; Fiber: 7.6g

372. **Gobi Masala Soup**

Servings: 4,

Cooking Time: 35 minutes

INGREDIENTS

- 1 tsp salt
- 1 tsp ground turmeric
- 1 tsp ground coriander
- 2 tsp cumin seeds
- 3 tsp dark mustard seeds
- 1 cup water
- 3 cups beef broth

- 1 head cauliflower, chopped
- 3 carrots, chopped
- 1 large onion, chopped
- 2 tbsp coconut oil
- Chopped cilantro for topping
- Crushed red pepper to taste
- Black pepper to taste
- 1 tbsp lemon juice

DIRECTIONS

1. On medium high fire, place a large heavy bottomed pot and heat coconut oil.
2. Once hot, sauté garlic cloves for a minute. Add carrots and continue sautéing for 4 minutes more.
3. Add turmeric, coriander, cumin, mustard seeds, and cauliflower. Sauté for 5 minutes.
4. Add water and beef broth and simmer for 10 to 15 minutes.
5. Turn off fire and transfer to blender. Puree until smoot and creamy.
6. Return to pot, continue simmering for another ten minutes.
7. Season with crushed red pepper, lemon juice, pepper, and salt.
8. To serve, garnish with cilantro, and enjoy.

NUTRITION: Calories: 148; Carbs: 16.1g; Protein: 3.7g; Fat: 8.8g

373. Greek Styled Veggie-Rice

Servings: 6,

Cooking Time: 20 minutes

INGREDIENTS

- pepper and salt to taste
- ¼ cup extra virgin olive oil
- 3 tbsp chopped fresh mint
- ½ cup grape tomatoes, halved
- ½ red bell pepper, diced small
- 1 head cauliflower, cut into large florets
- ¼ cup fresh lemon juice
- ½ yellow onion, minced

DIRECTIONS

1. In a bowl mix lemon juice and onion and leave for 30 minutes. Then drain onion and reserve the juice and onion bits.
2. In a blender, shred cauliflower until the size of a grain of rice.
3. On medium fire, place a medium nonstick skillet and for 8-10 minutes cook cauliflower while covered.
4. Add grape tomatoes and bell pepper and cook for 3 minutes while stirring occasionally.
5. Add mint and onion bits. Cook for another three minutes.
6. Meanwhile, in a small bowl whisk pepper, salt, 3 tbsp reserved lemon juice and olive oil until well blended.
7. Remove cooked cauliflower, transfer to a serving bowl, pour lemon juice mixture and toss to mix.
8. Before serving, if needed season with pepper and salt to taste.

NUTRITION:Calories: 120; Carbs: 8.0g; Protein: 2.3g; Fat: 9.5g

374. Green Vegan Soup

Servings: 6,

Cooking Time: 20 minutes

INGREDIENTS

- 1 medium head cauliflower, cut into bite-sized florets
- 1 medium white onion, peeled and diced
- 2 cloves garlic, peeled and diced
- 1 bay leaf crumbled
- 5-oz watercress
- fresh spinach or frozen spinach
- 1-liter vegetable stock or bone broth
- 1 cup cream or coconut milk + 6 tbsp for garnish
- 1/4 cup ghee or coconut oil
- 1 tsp salt or to taste
- freshly ground black pepper
- Optional: fresh herbs such as parsley or chives for garnish

DIRECTIONS

1. On medium-high the fire, place a Dutch oven greased with ghee. Once hot, sauté garlic for a minute. Add onions and sauté until soft and translucent, about 5 minutes.
2. Add cauliflower florets and crumbled bay leaf. Mix well and cook for 5 minutes.
3. Stir in watercress and spinach. Sauté for 3 minutes.
4. Add vegetable stock and bring to a boil.

5. When cauliflower is crisp-tender, stir in coconut milk.
6. Season with pepper and salt.
7. With a hand blender, puree soup until smooth and creamy.
8. Serve and enjoy.

NUTRITION:Calories: 392; Protein: 4.9g; Carbs: 9.7g; Sugar: 6.8g; Fat: 37.6g

375. Grilled Eggplant Caprese

Servings: 4,

Cooking Time: 10 minutes

INGREDIENTS

- 1 eggplant aubergine, small/medium
- 1 tomato large
- 2 basil leaves or a little more as needed
- 4-oz mozzarella
- good quality olive oil
- Pepper and salt to taste

DIRECTIONS

1. Cut the ends of the eggplant and then cut it lengthwise into ¼-inch thick slices. Discard the smaller pieces that's mostly skin and short.
2. Slice the tomatoes and mozzarella into thin slices just like the eggplant.
3. On medium-high the fire, place a griddle and let it heat up.
4. Brush eggplant slices with olive oil and place on grill. Grill for 3 minutes. Turnover and grill for a minute. Add a slice of cheese on one side and tomato on the other side. Continue cooking for another 2 minutes.
5. Sprinkle with basil leaves. Season with pepper and salt.

6. Fold eggplant in half and skewer with a cocktail stick.
7. Serve and enjoy.

NUTRITION:Calories: 59; Protein: 3.0g; Carbs: 4.0g; Sugar: 2.0g; Fat: 3.0g

376. Grilled Zucchini Bread and Cheese Sandwich

Servings: 2,

Cooking Time: 40 minutes

INGREDIENTS

- 1 large egg
- 1/2 cup freshly grated Parmesan
- 1/4 cup almond flour
- 2 cup grated zucchini
- 2 cup shredded Cheddar
- 2 green onions thinly sliced
- Freshly ground black pepper
- kosher salt
- Vegetable oil, for cooking

DIRECTIONS

1. With a paper towel, squeeze dry the zucchinis and place in a bowl. Add almond flour, green onions, Parmesan, and egg. Season with pepper and salt. Whisk well to combine.
2. Place a large nonstick pan on medium the fire and add oil to cover pan. Once hot, add ¼ cup of zucchini mixture and shape into a square like a bread. Add another batch as many as you can put in the pan. If needed, cook in batches. Cook for four minutes per side and place on a paper towel lined plate.
3. Once done cooking zucchinis, wipe off oil from the pan. Place one zucchini

piece on the pan, spread ½ of shredded cheese, and then top with another piece of zucchini. Grill for two minutes per side. Repeat process to make 2 sandwiches.

4. Serve and enjoy.

NUTRITION: Calories: 667; Protein: 41.5g; Carbs: 14.4g; Fat: 49.9g

377. <u>Hoemade Egg Drop Soup</u>

Servings: 4,

Cooking Time: 15 minutes

INGREDIENTS

- 1 tbsp cornstarch
- 1 tbsp dried minced onion
- 1 tsp dried parsley
- 2 eggs
- 4 cubes chicken bouillon
- 4 cups water
- 1 cup chopped carrots
- ½ cup thinly shredded cabbage

DIRECTIONS

1. Combine water, bouillon, parsley, cabbage, carrots, and onion flakes in a saucepan, and then bring to a boil.
2. Beat the eggs lightly and stir into the soup.
3. Dissolve cornstarch with a little water. Stir until smooth and stir into the soup. Let it boil until the soup thickens.

NUTRITION: Calories: 98; Carbs: 6.9g; Protein: 5.1g; Fat: 5.3g

378. <u>Hot and Sour Soup</u>

Servings: 4,

Cooking Time: 25 minutes

INGREDIENTS

- ½ tsp sesame oil
- 1 cup fresh bean sprouts
- 1 egg, lightly beaten
- 1 tsp black pepper
- 1 tsp ground ginger
- 3 tbsp white vinegar
- 3 tbsp soy sauce
- ¼ lb. sliced mushrooms
- ½ lb. tofu, cubed
- 2 tbsp corn starch
- 3 ½ cups chicken broth

DIRECTIONS

1. Mix corn starch and ¼ cup chicken broth and put aside.
2. Over high heat place a pot then combine and boil: pepper, ginger, vinegar, soy sauce, mushrooms, tofu and chicken broth.
3. Once boiling, add the corn starch mixture. Stir constantly and reduce fire. Once concoction is thickened, drop the slightly beaten egg while stirring vigorously.
4. Add bean sprouts and for one to two minutes allow simmering.
5. Remove from fire and transfer to serving bowls and enjoy while hot.

NUTRITION: Calories: 141; Carbs: 12.9g; Protein: 10.0g; Fat: 6.6g

379. Indian Bell Peppers and Potato Stir Fry

Servings: 2,

Cooking Time: 15 minutes

INGREDIENTS

- 1 tablespoon oil
- ½ teaspoon cumin seeds
- 4 cloves of garlic, minced
- 4 potatoes, scrubbed and halved
- Salt and pepper to taste
- 5 tablespoons water
- 2 bell peppers, seeded and julienned
- Chopped cilantro for garnish

DIRECTIONS

1. Heat oil in a skillet over medium flame and toast the cumin seeds until fragrant.
2. Add the garlic until fragrant.
3. Stir in the potatoes, salt, pepper, water, and bell peppers.
4. Close the lid and allow to simmer for at least 10 minutes.
5. Garnish with cilantro before cooking time ends.
6. Place in individual containers.
7. Put a label and store in the fridge.
8. Allow to thaw at room temperature before heating in the microwave oven.

NUTRITION: Calories: 83; Carbs: 7.3g; Protein: 2.8g; Fat: 6.4g; Fiber:1.7 g

380. Indian Style Okra

Servings: 4,

Cooking Time: 12 minutes

INGREDIENTS

- 1 lb. small to medium okra pods, trimmed
- ¼ tsp curry powder
- ½ tsp kosher salt
- 1 tsp finely chopped serrano chile
- 1 tsp ground coriander
- 1 tbsp canola oil
- ¾ tsp brown mustard seeds

DIRECTIONS

1. On medium high fire, place a large and heavy skillet and cook mustard seeds until fragrant, around 30 seconds.
2. Add canola oil. Add okra, curry powder, salt, chile, and coriander. Sauté for a minute while stirring every once in a while.
3. Cover and cook low fire for at least 8 minutes. Stir occasionally.
4. Uncover, increase fire to medium high and cook until okra is lightly browned, around 2 minutes more.
5. Serve and enjoy.

NUTRITION: Calories: 78; Carbs: 6.4g; Protein: 2.1g; Fat: 5.7g

381. Instant Pot Artichoke Hearts

Servings: 6,

Cooking Time: 30 minutes

INGREDIENTS

- 4 artichokes, rinsed and trimmed
- Juice from 2 small lemons, freshly squeezed
- 2 cups bone broth
- 1 tablespoon tarragon leaves
- 1 stalk, celery
- ½ cup extra virgin olive oil
- Salt and pepper to taste

DIRECTIONS

1. Place all ingredients in a pressure cooker.
2. Give a good stir.
3. Close the lid and seal the valve.
4. Pressure cook for 4 minutes.
5. Allow pressure cooker to release steam naturally.
6. Then serve and enjoy.

NUTRITION: Calories: 133; Carbs: 14.3g; Protein: 4.4g; Fat: 11.7g

382. **Instant Pot Fried Veggies**

Servings: 3,

Cooking Time: 6 minutes

INGREDIENTS

- 1 tablespoon olive oil
- 1 onion, chopped
- 4 cloves of garlic, minced
- 2 carrots, peeled and julienned
- 1 zucchini, julienned
- 1 large potato, peeled and julienned
- ½ cup chopped tomatoes
- 1 teaspoon rosemary sprig
- Salt and pepper to taste

Instructions

1. Press the Sauté button and heat the oil.
2. Sauté the onion and garlic until fragrant.
3. Stir in the rest of the ingredients.
4. Close the lid and make sure that the vents are sealed.
5. Press the Manual button and adjust the cooking time to 1 minute.
6. Do quick pressure release.
7. Once the lid is open, press the Sauté button and continue stirring until the liquid has reduced.
8. Once cooled, evenly divide into serving size, keep in your preferred container, and refrigerate until ready to eat.

NUTRITION: Calories: 97; Carbs: 10.4g; Protein: 0.5g; Fat: 4.2g

383. **Instant Pot Sautéed Kale**

Servings: 6,

Cooking Time: minutes

INGREDIENTS

- 3 tablespoons coconut oil
- 2 cloves of garlic, minced
- 1 onion, chopped
- 2 teaspoons crushed red pepper flakes
- 4cups kale, chopped
- ¼ cup water
- Salt and pepper to taste

DIRECTIONS

1. Press the "Sauté" button on the Instant Pot.
2. Heat the oil and sauté the garlic and onions until fragrant.

3. Stir in the rest of the ingredients.

4. Close the lid and make sure that the steam release valve is set to "Sealing."

5. Press the "Manual" button and adjust the cooking time to 4 minutes.

6. Do quick pressure release.

NUTRITION: Calories: 82; Carbs: 5.1g; Protein: 1.1g; Fat: 7.9g

BREADS AND PIZZA

384. Fig Relish Panini

Servings: 4

Cooking Time: 40 minutes

INGREDIENTS

- Grated parmesan cheese, for garnish
- Olive oil
- Fig relish (recipe follows)
- Arugula
- Basil leaves
- Toma cheese, grated or sliced
- Sweet butter
- 4 ciabatta slices

Fig Relish INGREDIENTS

- 1 tsp dry mustard
- Pinch of salt
- 1 tsp mustard seed
- ½ cup apple cider vinegar
- ½ cup sugar
- ½ lb. Mission figs, stemmed and peeled

DIRECTIONS

1. Create fig relish by mincing the figs. Then put in all ingredients, except for the dry mustard, in a small pot and simmer for 30 minutes until it becomes jam like. Season with dry mustard according to taste and let cool before refrigerating.
2. Spread sweet butter on two slices of ciabatta rolls and layer on the following: cheese, basil leaves, arugula and fig relish then cover with the remaining bread slice.
3. Grill in a Panini press until cheese is melted and bread is crisped and ridged.

NUTRITION:Calories: 264; Carbs: 55.1g; Protein: 6.0g; Fat: 4.2g

385. Fruity and Cheesy Quesadilla

Servings: 1,

Cooking Time: 15 minutes

INGREDIENTS

- ¼ cup hand grated jack cheese
- ½ cup finely chopped fresh mango
- 1 large whole-grain tortilla
- 1 tbsp chopped fresh cilantro

DIRECTIONS

1. In a medium bowl, mix cilantro and mango.
2. Place mango mixture inside tortilla and top with cheese.
3. Pop in a preheated 350oF oven and bake until cheese is melted completely around 10 to 15 minutes.

NUTRITION:Calories: 169; Fat: 9g; Protein: 7g; Carbohydrates: 15g

386. Garlic & Tomato Gluten Free Focaccia

Servings: 8,

Cooking Time: 20 minutes

INGREDIENTS

- 1 egg
- ½ tsp lemon juice
- 1 tbsp honey
- 4 tbsp olive oil
- A pinch of sugar
- 1 ¼ cup warm water
- 1 tbsp active dry yeast
- 2 tsp rosemary, chopped
- 2 tsp thyme, chopped
- 2 tsp basil, chopped
- 2 cloves garlic, minced
- 1 ¼ tsp sea salt
- 2 tsp xanthan gum
- ½ cup millet flour
- 1 cup potato starch, not flour
- 1 cup sorghum flour
- Gluten free cornmeal for dusting

DIRECTIONS

1. For 5 minutes, turn on the oven and then turn it off, while keeping oven door closed.
2. In a small bowl, mix warm water and pinch of sugar. Add yeast and swirl gently. Leave for 7 minutes.
3. In a large mixing bowl, whisk well herbs, garlic, salt, xanthan gum, starch, and flours.
4. Once yeast is done proofing, pour into bowl of flours. Whisk in egg, lemon juice, honey, and olive oil.
5. Mix thoroughly and place in a well-greased square pan, dusted with cornmeal.
6. Top with fresh garlic, more herbs, and sliced tomatoes.
7. Place in the warmed oven and let it rise for half an hour.

8. Turn on oven to 375oF and after preheating time it for 20 minutes. Focaccia is done once tops are lightly browned.
9. Remove from oven and pan immediately and let it cool.
10. Best served when warm.

NUTRITION: Calories: 251; Carbs: 38.4g; Protein: 5.4g; Fat: 9.0g

387. Garlic-Rosemary Dinner Rolls

Servings: 8,

Cooking Time: 20 minutes

INGREDIENTS

- 2 garlic cloves, minced
- 1 tsp dried crushed rosemary
- ½ tsp apple cider vinegar
- 2 tbsp olive oil
- 2 eggs
- 1 ¼ tsp salt
- 1 ¾ tsp xanthan gum
- ½ cup tapioca starch
- ¾ cup brown rice flour
- 1 cup sorghum flour
- 2 tsp dry active yeast
- 1 tbsp honey
- ¾ cup hot water

DIRECTIONS

1. Mix well water and honey in a small bowl and add yeast. Leave it for exactly 7 minutes.
2. In a large bowl, mix the following with a paddle mixer: garlic, rosemary, salt, xanthan gum, sorghum flour, tapioca starch, and brown rice flour.

3. In a medium bowl, whisk well vinegar, olive oil, and eggs.
4. Into bowl of dry ingredients pour in vinegar and yeast mixture and mix well.
5. Grease a 12-muffin tin with cooking spray. Transfer dough evenly into 12 muffin tins and leave it 20 minutes to rise.
6. Then preheat oven to 375oF and bake dinner rolls until tops are golden brown, around 17 to 19 minutes.
7. Remove dinner rolls from oven and muffin tins immediately and let it cool.
8. Best served when warm.

NUTRITION: Calories: 200; Carbs: 34.3g; Protein: 4.2g; Fat: 5.4g

388. <u>Grilled Burgers with Mushrooms</u>

Servings: 4,

Cooking Time: 10 minutes

INGREDIENTS

- 2 Bibb lettuce, halved
- 4 slices red onion
- 4 slices tomato
- 4 whole wheat buns, toasted
- 2 tbsp olive oil
- ¼ tsp cayenne pepper, optional
- 1 garlic clove, minced
- 1 tbsp sugar
- ½ cup water
- 1/3 cup balsamic vinegar
- 4 large Portobello mushroom caps, around 5-inches in diameter

DIRECTIONS

1. Remove stems from mushrooms and clean with a damp cloth. Transfer into a baking dish with gill-side up.
2. In a bowl, mix thoroughly olive oil, cayenne pepper, garlic, sugar, water and vinegar. Pour over mushrooms and marinate mushrooms in the ref for at least an hour.
3. Once the one hour is nearly up, preheat grill to medium high fire and grease grill grate.
4. Grill mushrooms for five minutes per side or until tender. Baste mushrooms with marinade so it doesn't dry up.
5. To assemble, place ½ of bread bun on a plate, top with a slice of onion, mushroom, tomato and one lettuce leaf. Cover with the other top half of the bun. Repeat process with remaining ingredients, serve and enjoy.

NUTRITION: Calories: 244.1; Carbs: 32g; Protein: 8.1g; Fat: 9.3g

389. <u>Grilled Sandwich with Goat Cheese</u>

Servings: 4

Cooking Time: 8 minutes

INGREDIENTS

- ½ cup soft goat cheese
- 4 Kaiser rolls 2-oz
- ¼ tsp freshly ground black pepper
- ¼ tsp salt
- 1/3 cup chopped basil
- Cooking spray
- 4 big Portobello mushroom caps

- 1 yellow bell pepper, cut in half and seeded
- 1 red bell pepper, cut in half and seeded
- 1 garlic clove, minced
- 1 tbsp olive oil
- ¼ cup balsamic vinegar

DIRECTIONS

1. In a large bowl, mix garlic, olive oil and balsamic vinegar. Add mushroom and bell peppers. Gently mix to coat. Remove veggies from vinegar and discard vinegar mixture.
2. Coat with cooking spray a grill rack and the grill preheated to medium high fire.
3. Place mushrooms and bell peppers on the grill and grill for 4 minutes per side. Remove from grill and let cool a bit.
4. Into thin strips, cut the bell peppers.
5. In a small bowl, combine black pepper, salt, basil and sliced bell peppers.
6. Horizontally, cut the Kaiser rolls and evenly spread cheese on the cut side. Arrange 1 Portobello per roll, top with 1/3 bell pepper mixture and cover with the other half of the roll.
7. Grill the rolls as you press down on them to create a Panini like line on the bread. Grill until bread is toasted.

NUTRITION: Calories: 317; Carbs: 41.7g; Protein: 14.0g; Fat: 10.5g

390. Halibut Sandwiches Mediterranean Style

Servings: 4

Cooking Time: 23 minutes

196

INGREDIENTS

- 2 packed cups arugula or 2 oz.
- Grated zest of 1 large lemon
- 1 tbsp capers, drained and mashed
- 2 tbsp fresh flat leaf parsley, chopped
- ¼ cup fresh basil, chopped
- ¼ cup sun dried tomatoes, chopped
- ¼ cup reduced fat mayonnaise
- 1 garlic clove, halved
- 1 pc of 14 oz of ciabatta loaf bread with ends trimmed and split in half, horizontally
- 2 tbsp plus 1 tsp olive oil, divided
- Kosher salt and freshly ground pepper
- 2 pcs or 6 oz halibut fillets, skinned
- Cooking spray

DIRECTIONS

1. Heat oven to 450oF.
2. With cooking spray, coat a baking dish. Season halibut with a pinch of pepper and salt plus rub with a tsp of oil and place on baking dish. Then put in oven and bake until cooked or for ten to fifteen minutes. Remove from oven and let cool.
3. Get a slice of bread and coat with olive oil the sliced portions. Put in oven and cook until golden, around six to eight minutes. Remove from heat and rub garlic on the bread.
4. Combine the following in a medium bowl: lemon zest, capers, parsley, basil, sun dried tomatoes and mayonnaise. Then add the halibut, mashing with fork until flaked. Spread the mixture on one side of bread, add arugula and cover with the other bread half and serve.

NUTRITION: Calories: 125; Carbs: 8.0g; Protein: 3.9g; Fat: 9.2g

391. Herbed Panini Fillet O'Fish

Servings: 4

Cooking Time: 25 minutes

INGREDIENTS

- 4 slices thick sourdough bread
- 4 slices mozzarella cheese
- 1 portabella mushroom, sliced
- 1 small onion, sliced
- 6 tbsp oil
- 4 garlic and herb fish fillets

DIRECTIONS

1. Prepare your fillets by adding salt, pepper and herbs (rosemary, thyme, parsley whatever you like). Then dredged in flour before deep frying in very hot oil. Once nicely browned, remove from oil and set aside.
2. On medium high fire, sauté for five minutes the onions and mushroom in a skillet with 2 tbsp oil.
3. Prepare sourdough breads by layering the following over it: cheese, fish fillet, onion mixture and cheese again before covering with another bread slice.
4. Grill in your Panini press until cheese is melted and bread is crisped and ridged.

NUTRITION: Calories: 422; Carbs: 13.2g; Protein: 51.2g; Fat: 17.2g

392. Italian Flat Bread Gluten Free

Servings: 8,

Cooking Time: 30 minutes

INGREDIENTS

- 1 tbsp apple cider
- 2 tbsp water
- ½ cup yogurt
- 2 tbsp butter
- 2 tbsp sugar
- 2 eggs
- 1 tsp xanthan gum
- ½ tsp salt
- 1 tsp baking soda
- 1 ½ tsp baking powder
- ½ cup potato starch, not potato flour
- ½ cup tapioca flour
- ¼ cup brown rice flour
- 1/3 cup sorghum flour

DIRECTIONS

1. With parchment paper, line an 8 x 8-inch baking pan and grease parchment paper. Preheat oven to 375oF.
2. Mix xanthan gum, salt, baking soda, baking powder, all flours, and starch in a large bowl.
3. Whisk well sugar and eggs in a medium bowl until creamed. Add vinegar, water, yogurt, and butter. Whisk thoroughly.
4. Pour in egg mixture into bowl of flours and mix well.
5. Transfer sticky dough into prepared pan and bake in the oven for 25 to 30 minutes.

6. If tops of bread start to brown a lot, cover top with foil and continue baking until done.
7. Remove from oven and pan right away and let it cool.
8. Best served when warm.

NUTRITION:Calories: 166; Carbs: 27.8g; Protein: 3.4g; Fat: 4.8g

393. Lemon Aioli and Swordfish Panini

Servings: 4

Cooking Time: 25 minutes

Swordfish Panini INGREDIENTS

- 2 oz fresh arugula greens
- 1 loaf focaccia bread
- 2 cloves garlic minced
- 1 tbsp herbes de Provence
- Pepper and salt
- 4 pcs of 6oz swordfish fillet
- 1 ½ tbsp olive oil

Lemon Aioli INGREDIENTS

- ¼ tsp freshly ground black pepper
- ¼ tsp salt
- 1 clove garlic, minced
- 2 tbsp fresh lemon juice
- 1 lemon, zested
- 2/3 cup mayonnaise

DIRECTIONS

1. In a small bowl, mix well all lemon Aioli ingredients and put aside.
2. Over medium high fire, heat olive oil in skillet. Season with pepper, salt, minced garlic and herbs de Provence the swordfish. Then pan fry fish until

golden brown on both sides, around 5 minutes per side.
3. Slice bread into four slices. Smear on the lemon aioli mixture on two bread slices, layer with arugula leaves and fried fish then cover with the remaining bread slices before grilling in a Panini press.
4. Grill until bread is crisped and ridged.

NUTRITION:Calories: 433; Carbs: 15.0g; Protein: 36.2g; Fat: 25.1g

394. Lemon, Buttered Shrimp Panini

Servings: 4

Cooking Time: 10 minutes

INGREDIENTS

- 3 tbsp butter
- 1 baguette
- 1 tsp hot sauce
- 1 tbsp parsley
- 2 tbsp lemon juice
- 4 garlic cloves, minced
- 1 lb. shrimp peeled

DIRECTIONS

1. Make a hollowed portion on your baguette.
2. Sauté the following on a skillet with melted butter: parsley, hot sauce, lemon juice and garlic. After a minute or two mix in the shrimps and sautéing for five minutes.
3. Scoop shrimps into baguette and grill in a Panini press until baguette is crisped and ridged.

NUTRITION: Calories: 262; Carbs: 14.1g; Protein: 26.1g; Fat: 10.8g

395. <u>Mediterranean Baba Ghanoush</u>

Servings: 4

Cooking Time: 25 minutes

INGREDIENTS

- 1 bulb garlic
- 1 red bell pepper, halved and seeded
- 1 tbsp chopped fresh basil
- 1 tbsp olive oil
- 1 tsp black pepper
- 2 eggplants, sliced lengthwise
- 2 rounds of flatbread or pita
- Juice of 1 lemon

DIRECTIONS

1. Grease grill grate with cooking spray and preheat grill to medium high.
2. Slice tops of garlic bulb and wrap in foil. Place in the cooler portion of the grill and roast for at least 20 minutes.
3. Place bell pepper and eggplant slices on the hottest part of grill.
4. Grill for at least two to three minutes each side.
5. Once bulbs are done, peel off skins of roasted garlic and place peeled garlic into food processor.
6. Add olive oil, pepper, basil, lemon juice, grilled red bell pepper and grilled eggplant.
7. Puree until smooth and transfer into a bowl.
8. Grill bread at least 30 seconds per side to warm.
9. Serve bread with the pureed dip and enjoy.

NUTRITION: Calories: 213.6; Carbs: 36.3g; Protein: 6.3g; Fat: 4.8g

396. <u>Multi Grain & Gluten Free Dinner Rolls</u>

Servings: 8,

Cooking Time: 20 minutes

INGREDIENTS

- ½ tsp apple cider vinegar
- 3 tbsp olive oil
- 2 eggs
- 1 tsp baking powder
- 1 tsp salt
- 2 tsp xanthan gum
- ½ cup tapioca starch
- ¼ cup brown teff flour
- ¼ cup flax meal
- ¼ cup amaranth flour
- ¼ cup sorghum flour
- ¾ cup brown rice flour

DIRECTIONS

1. Mix well water and honey in a small bowl and add yeast. Leave it for exactly 10 minutes.
2. In a large bowl, mix the following with a paddle mixer: baking powder, salt, xanthan gum, flax meal, sorghum flour, teff flour, tapioca starch, amaranth flour, and brown rice flour.
3. In a medium bowl, whisk well vinegar, olive oil, and eggs.
4. Into bowl of dry ingredients pour in vinegar and yeast mixture and mix well.
5. Grease a 12-muffin tin with cooking spray. Transfer dough evenly into 12

muffin tins and leave it for an hour to rise.

6. Then preheat oven to 375oF and bake dinner rolls until tops are golden brown, around 20 minutes.

7. Remove dinner rolls from oven and muffin tins immediately and let it cool.

8. Best served when warm.

NUTRITION:Calories: 207; Carbs: 28.4g; Protein: 4.6g; Fat: 8.3g

397. Mushroom and Eggplant Vegan Panini

Servings: 4

Cooking Time: 18 minutes

INGREDIENTS

- 4 thin slices Asiago Cheese
- 4 thin slices Swiss cheese
- ¼ cup fat free ranch dressing
- 8 slices focaccia bread
- 2 tsp grated parmesan cheese
- 1 tsp onion powder
- 1 tsp garlic powder
- 4 slices ½-inch thick eggplant, peeled
- 1 cup fat-free balsamic vinaigrette
- 4 portobello mushroom caps
- 2 red bell peppers

DIRECTIONS

1. Broil peppers in oven for five minutes or until its skin has blistered and blackened. Remove peppers and place in bowl while quickly covering with plastic wrap, let cool for twenty minutes before peeling off the skin and refrigerating overnight.

2. In a re-sealable bag, place mushrooms and vinaigrette and marinate in the ref for a night.

3. Next day, grill mushrooms while discarding marinade. While seasoning eggplant with onion and garlic powder then grill along with mushrooms until tender, around four to five minutes.

4. Remove mushrooms and eggplant from griller and top with parmesan.

5. On four slices of focaccia, smear ranch dressing evenly then layer: cheese, mushroom, roasted peppers and eggplant slices and cover with the remaining focaccia slices.

6. Grill in a Panini press until cheese has melted and bread is crisped and ridged.

NUTRITION:Calories: 574; Carbs: 77.1g; Protein: 29.6g; Fat: 19.9g

398. Open Face Egg and Bacon Sandwich

Servings: 1,

Cooking Time: 20 minutes

INGREDIENTS

- ¼ oz reduced fat cheddar, shredded
- ½ small jalapeno, thinly sliced
- ½ whole grain English muffin, split
- 1 large organic egg
- 1 thick slice of tomato
- 1-piece turkey bacon
- 2 thin slices red onion
- 4-5 sprigs fresh cilantro
- Cooking spray
- Pepper to taste

DIRECTIONS

1. On medium fire, place a skillet, cook bacon until crisp tender and set aside.
2. In same skillet, drain oils, and place ½ of English muffin and heat for at least a minute per side. Transfer muffin to a serving plate.
3. Coat the same skillet with cooking spray and fry egg to desired doneness. Once cooked, place egg on top of muffin.
4. Add cilantro, tomato, onion, jalapeno and bacon on top of egg. Serve and enjoy.

NUTRITION: Calories: 245; Carbs: 24.7g; Protein: 11.8g; Fat: 11g

399. **Paleo Chocolate Banana Bread**

Servings: 10,

Cooking Time: 50 minutes

INGREDIENTS

- ¼ cup dark chocolate, chopped
- ½ cup almond butter
- ½ cup coconut flour, sifted
- ½ teaspoon cinnamon powder
- 1 teaspoon baking soda
- 1 teaspoon vanilla extract
- 4 bananas, mashed
- 4 eggs
- 4 tablespoon coconut oil, melted
- A pinch of salt

DIRECTIONS

1. Preheat the oven to 350oF.
2. Grease an 8" x 8" square pan and set aside.

3. In a large bowl, mix together the eggs, banana, vanilla extract, almond butter and coconut oil. Mix well until well combined.
4. Add the cinnamon powder, coconut flour, baking powder, baking soda and salt to the wet ingredients. Fold until well combined. Add in the chopped chocolates then fold the batter again.
5. Pour the batter into the greased pan. Spread evenly.
6. Bake in the oven for about 50 minutes or until a toothpick inserted in the center comes out clean.
7. Remove from the hot oven and cool in a wire rack for an hour.

NUTRITION: Calories: 150.3; Carbs: 13.9g; Protein: 3.2g; Fat: 9.1g

400. **Panini and Eggplant Caponata**

Servings: 4

Cooking Time: 10 minutes

INGREDIENTS

- ¼ cup packed fresh basil leaves
- ¼ of a 7oz can of eggplant caponata
- 4 oz thinly sliced mozzarella
- 1 tbsp olive oil
- 1 ciabatta roll 6-7-inch length, horizontally split

DIRECTIONS

1. Spread oil evenly on the sliced part of the ciabatta and layer on the following: cheese, caponata, basil leaves and cheese again before covering with another slice of ciabatta.

2. Then grill sandwich in a Panini press until cheese melts and bread gets crisped and ridged.

NUTRITION: Calories: 295; Carbs: 44.4g; Protein: 16.4g; Fat: 7.3g

401. Panini with Chicken-Fontina

Servings: 2,

Cooking Time: 45 minutes

INGREDIENTS

- ¼ Cup Arugula
- 2 oz sliced cooked chicken
- 3 oz fontina cheese thinly sliced
- 1 tbsp Dijon mustard
- 1 ciabatta roll
- ¼ cup water
- 1 tbsp + 1 tsp olive oil
- 1 large onion, diced

DIRECTIONS

1. On medium low fire, place a skillet and heat 1 tbsp oil. Sauté onion and cook for 5 minutes. Pour in water while stirring and cooking continuously for 30 minutes until onion is golden brown and tender.
2. Slice bread roll lengthwise and spread the following on one bread half, on the cut side: mustard, caramelized onion, chicken, arugula and cheese. Cover with the remaining bread half.
3. Place the sandwich in a Panini maker and grill for 5 to 8 minutes or until cheese is melted and bread is ridged and crisped.

NUTRITION: Calories: 216; Carbs: 18.7g; Protein: 22.3g; Fat: 24.5g

402. Pesto, Avocado and Tomato Panini

Servings: 4

Cooking Time: 10 minutes

Panini INGREDIENTS

- 2 tbsp extra virgin olive oil
- 8 oz fresh buffalo mozzarella cheese
- 2 vine-ripened tomatoes cut into ¼ inch thick slices
- 2 avocados, peeled, pitted, quartered and cut into thin strips
- 1 ciabatta loaf

Pesto INGREDIENTS

- Pepper and salt
- ½ lemon
- 1/3 cup extra virgin olive oil
- 1/3 cup parmesan cheese
- 1/3 cup pine nuts, toasted
- 1 ½ bunches fresh basil leaves
- 2 garlic cloves, peeled

DIRECTIONS

1. To make the pesto, puree garlic in a food processor and transfer to a mortar and pestle and add in basil and smash into a coarse paste like consistency. Mix in the pine nuts and continue crushing. Once paste like, add the parmesan cheese and mix. Pour in olive oil and blend thoroughly while adding lemon juice. Season with pepper and salt. Put aside.
2. Prepare Panini by slicing ciabatta loaf in three horizontal pieces. To prepare

Panini, over bottom loaf slice layer the following: avocado, tomato, pepper, salt and mozzarella cheese. Then top with the middle ciabatta slice and repeat layering process again and cover with the topmost ciabatta bread slice.
3. Grill in a Panini press until cheese is melted and bred is crisped and ridged.

NUTRITION: Calories: 577; Carbs: 15.5g; Protein: 24.2g; Fat: 49.3g

403. Quinoa Pizza Muffins

Servings: 4

Cooking Time: 30 minutes

INGREDIENTS

- 1 cup uncooked quinoa
- 2 large eggs
- ½ medium onion, diced
- 1 cup diced bell pepper
- 1 cup shredded mozzarella cheese
- 1 tbsp dried basil
- 1 tbsp dried oregano
- 2 tsp garlic powder
- 1/8 tsp salt
- 1 tsp crushed red peppers
- ½ cup roasted red pepper, chopped*
- Pizza Sauce, about 1-2 cups

DIRECTIONS

1. Preheat oven to 350oF.
2. Cook quinoa according to directions.
3. Combine all ingredients (except sauce) into bowl. Mix all ingredients well.
4. Scoop quinoa pizza mixture into muffin tin evenly. Makes 12 muffins.

5. Bake for 30 minutes until muffins turn golden in color and the edges are getting crispy.
6. Top with 1 or 2 tbsp pizza sauce and enjoy!

NUTRITION: Calories: 303; Carbs: 41.3g; Protein: 21.0g; Fat: 6.1g

404. Rosemary-Walnut Loaf Bread

Servings: 8,

Cooking Time: 45 minutes

INGREDIENTS

- ½ cup chopped walnuts
- 4 tbsp fresh, chopped rosemary
- 1 1/3 cups lukewarm carbonated water
- 1 tbsp honey
- ½ cup extra virgin olive oil
- 1 tsp apple cider vinegar
- 3 eggs
- 5 tsp instant dry yeast granules
- 1 tsp salt
- 1 tbsp xanthan gum
- ¼ cup buttermilk powder
- 1 cup white rice flour
- 1 cup tapioca starch
- 1 cup arrowroot starch
- 1 ¼ cups all-purpose Bob's Red Mill gluten-free flour mix

DIRECTIONS

1. In a large mixing bowl, whisk well eggs. Add 1 cup warm water, honey, olive oil, and vinegar.

2. While beating continuously, add the rest of the ingredients except for rosemary and walnuts.
3. Continue beating. If dough is too stiff, add a bit of warm water. Dough should be shaggy and thick.
4. Then add rosemary and walnuts continue kneading until evenly distributed.
5. Cover bowl of dough with a clean towel, place in a warm spot, and let it rise for 30 minutes.
6. Fifteen minutes into rising time, preheat oven to 400oF.
7. Generously grease with olive oil a 2-quart Dutch oven and preheat inside oven without the lid.
8. Once dough is done rising, remove pot from oven, and place dough inside. With a wet spatula, spread top of dough evenly in pot.
9. Brush tops of bread with 2 tbsp of olive oil, cover Dutch oven and bake for 35 to 45 minutes.
10. Once bread is done, remove from oven. And gently remove bread from pot.
11. Allow bread to cool at least ten minutes before slicing.
12. Serve and enjoy.

NUTRITION: Calories: 424; Carbs: 56.8g; Protein: 7.0g; Fat: 19.0g

405. Sandwich with Hummus

Servings: 4

Cooking Time: 0 minutes

INGREDIENTS

- 4 cups alfalfa sprouts
- 1 cup cucumber sliced 1/8 inch thick
- 4 red onion sliced ¼-inch thick
- 8 tomatoes sliced ¼-inch thick
- 2 cups shredded Bibb lettuce
- 12 slices 1-oz whole wheat bread
- 1 can 15.5-oz chickpeas, drained
- 2 garlic cloves, peeled
- ¼ tsp salt
- ½ tsp ground cumin
- 1 tbsp tahini
- 1 tbsp lemon juice
- 2 tbsp water
- 3 tbsp plain fat free yogurt

DIRECTIONS

1. In a food processor, blend chickpeas, garlic, salt, cumin, tahini, lemon juice, water and yogurt until smooth to create hummus.
2. On 1 slice of bread, spread 2 tbsp hummus, top with 1 onion slice, 2 tomato slices, ½ cup lettuce, another bread slice, 1 cup sprouts, ¼ cup cucumber and cover with another bread slice. Repeat procedure for the rest of the ingredients.

NUTRITION: Calories: 407; Carbs: 67.7g; Protein: 18.8 g; Fat: 6.8g

406. Sandwich with Spinach and Tuna Salad

Servings: 4

Cooking Time: 0 minutes

INGREDIENTS

- 1 cup fresh baby spinach
- 8 slices 100% whole wheat sandwich bread
- ¼ tsp freshly ground black pepper

- ½ tsp salt free seasoning blend
- Juice of one lemon
- 2 tbsp olive oil
- ½ tsp dill weed
- 2 ribs celery, diced

DIRECTIONS

1. In a medium bowl, mix well dill weed, celery, onion, cucumber and tuna.
2. Add lemon juice and olive oil and mix thoroughly.
3. Season with pepper and salt-free seasoning blend.
4. To assemble sandwich, you can toast bread slices, on top of one bread slice layer ½ cup tuna salad, top with ¼ cup spinach and cover with another slice of bread.
5. Repeat procedure to remaining ingredients, serve and enjoy.

NUTRITION: Calories: 272.5; Carbs: 35.9g; Protein: 10.4g; Fat: 9.7g

407. **Spiced Roast Beef Panini**

Servings: 2,

Cooking Time: 15 minutes

INGREDIENTS

- Creamy horseradish sauce
- Butter
- 1 roasted red peppers
- 1 crusty bread, halved lengthwise
- 2 slices Havarti cheese
- 4 Slices deli roast beef

DIRECTIONS

1. On one bread slice, butter one side, spread over the horseradish sauce,

then add evenly the cheese and roast beef and topped with roasted peppers.
2. Cover the filling with the other bread half and start grilling in a Panini press for around three to five minutes while pressing down for a ridged effect.
3. Serve and enjoy.

NUTRITION: Calories: 311; Carbs: 33.8g; Protein: 17.3g; Fat: 11.7g

408. **Sun-Dried Tomatoes Panini**

Servings: 4,

Cooking Time: 15 minutes

INGREDIENTS

- ½ cup shredded mozzarella cheese
- 8 slices country style Italian bread
- 1/8 tsp freshly ground black pepper
- Cooking spray
- 3/8 tsp salt, divided
- 1 6oz package fresh baby spinach
- 8 garlic cloves, thinly sliced
- 1/8 tsp crushed red pepper
- ¼ cup chopped drained oil packed sun-dried tomato
- 4 4oz chicken cutlets
- 1 tsp chopped rosemary
- 2 tbsp extra virgin olive oil, divided

DIRECTIONS

1. In a re-sealable bag mix chicken, rosemary and 2 tsp olive oil. Allow to marinate for 30 minutes in the ref.
2. On medium high fire, place a skillet and heat 4 tsp oil. Sauté for a minute garlic, red pepper and sun-dried tomato. Add 1/8 tsp salt and spinach and cook for a minute and put aside.

3. On a grill pan coated with cooking spray, grill chicken for three minutes per side. Season with black pepper and salt.
4. To assemble the sandwich, evenly layer the following on one bread slice: cheese, spinach mixture, and chicken cutlet. Cover with another bread slice.
5. Place sandwich in a Panini press and grill for around five minutes or until cheese is melted and bread is crisped and ridged.

NUTRITION: Calories: 369; Carbs: 25.7g; Protein: 42.7g; Fat: 10.1g

409. Sunflower Gluten Free Bread

Servings: 8,

Cooking Time: 30 minutes

INGREDIENTS

- 1 tsp apple cider vinegar
- 3 tbsp olive oil
- 3 egg whites
- Extra seeds for sprinkling on top of loaf
- 1 ¼ tsp sea salt
- 2 ¾ tsp xanthan gum
- 2 tbsp hemp seeds
- 2 tbsp poppy seeds
- ¼ cup flax meal
- ¼ cup buckwheat flour
- ½ cup brown rice flour
- 1 cup tapioca starch
- 1 ½ cups sorghum flour
- 2 ½ tsp dry active yeast
- 1 tbsp honey
- 1 ¼ cup hot water

DIRECTIONS

1. Mix honey and water in a small bowl. Add yeast and stir a bit and leave on for 7 minutes.
2. In a large mixing bowl, mix well salt, xanthan gum, hemp, poppy, flax meal, buckwheat flour, brown rice four, tapioca starch, and sorghum flour and beat with a paddle mixer.
3. In a medium bowl, beat well vinegar, oil, and eggs.
4. In bowl of dry ingredients, pour in bowl of egg mixture and yeast mixture and mix well until you have a smooth dough.
5. In a greased 10-inch cast iron skillet, transfer dough. Lightly wet hands with warm water and smoothen surface of dough until the surface is even. (A 9-inch cake pan will also do nicely if you don't have a cast iron skillet).
6. Sprinkle extra seeds on top of dough and leave dough in a warm corner for 45 to 60 minutes to rise.
7. Then pop risen dough in a 375oF preheated oven until tops are golden brown, around 30 minutes.
8. Once done cooking, immediately remove dough from pan and let it cool a bit before slicing and serving.

NUTRITION: Calories: 291; Carbs: 49.1g; Protein: 6.0g; Fat: 8.5g

410. Tasty Crabby Panini

Servings: 4

Cooking Time: 10 minutes

INGREDIENTS

- 1 tbsp Olive oil

- French bread split and sliced diagonally
- 1 lb. blue crab meat or shrimp or spiny lobster or stone crab
- ½ cup celery
- ¼ cup green onion chopped
- 1 tsp Worcestershire sauce
- 1 tsp lemon juice
- 1 tbsp Dijon mustard
- ½ cup light mayonnaise

DIRECTIONS

1. In a medium bowl mix the following thoroughly: celery, onion, Worcestershire, lemon juice, mustard and mayonnaise. Season with pepper and salt. Then gently add in the almonds and crabs.
2. Spread olive oil on sliced sides of bread and smear with crab mixture before covering with another bread slice.
3. Grill sandwich in a Panini press until bread is crisped and ridged.

NUTRITION: Calories: 248; Carbs: 12.0g; Protein: 24.5g; Fat: 10.9g

411. **Tuna Melt Panini**

Servings: 4

Cooking Time: 10 minutes

INGREDIENTS

- 2 tbsp softened unsalted butter
- 16 pcs of 1/8-inch kosher dill pickle
- 8 pcs of ¼ inch thick cheddar or Swiss cheese
- Mayonnaise and Dijon mustard
- 4 ciabatta rolls, split
- Pepper and salt

- ½ tsp crushed red pepper
- 1 tbsp minced basil
- 1 tbsp balsamic vinegar
- ¼ cup extra virgin olive oil
- ¼ cup finely diced red onion
- 2 cans of 6oz albacore tuna

DIRECTIONS

1. Combine thoroughly the following in a bowl: salt pepper, crushed red pepper, basil, vinegar, olive oil, onion and tuna.
2. Smear with mayonnaise and mustard the cut sides of the bread rolls then layer on: cheese, tuna salad and pickles. Cover with the remaining slice of roll.
3. Grill in a Panini press ensuring that cheese is melted and bread is crisped and ridged.

NUTRITION: Calories: 539; Carbs: 27.7g; Protein: 21.6g; Fat: 38.5g

412. **Tuscan Bread Dipper**

Servings: 8,

Cooking Time: 0 minutes

INGREDIENTS

- ¼ cup balsamic vinegar
- ¼ cup extra virgin olive oil
- ¼ teaspoon salt
- ½ tbsp fresh basil, minced
- ½ teaspoon pepper
- 1 ½ teaspoon Italian seasoning
- 2 cloves garlic minced
- 8 pieces Food for Life Brown Rice English Muffins

DIRECTIONS

1. In a small bowl mix well all ingredients except for bread. Allow herbs to steep in olive oil-balsamic vinegar mixture for at least 30 minutes.
2. To serve, toast bread, cut each muffin in half and serve with balsamic vinegar dip.

NUTRITION: Calories: 168.5; Carbs: 27.7g; Protein: 5.2g; Fat: 4.1g

413. Keto Breakfast Pizza

Servings: 6

Preparation time: 30 mins

INGREDIENTS

- 2 tablespoons coconut flour
- 2 cups cauliflower, grated
- ½ teaspoon salt
- 1 tablespoon psyllium husk powder
- 4 eggs

Toppings:

- Avocado
- Smoked Salmon
- Herbs
- Olive oil
- Spinach

DIRECTIONS

1. Preheat the oven to 360 degrees and grease a pizza tray.
2. Mix together all ingredients in a bowl, except toppings, and keep aside.
3. Pour the pizza dough onto the pan and mold it into an even pizza crust using hands.

4. Top the pizza with toppings and transfer in the oven.
5. Bake for about 15 minutes until golden brown and remove from the oven to serve.

NUTRITION: Calories: 454 Carbs: 16g Fats: 31g Proteins: 22g Sodium: 1325mg Sugar: 4.4g

414. Coconut Flour Pizza

Servings: 4

Preparation time: 35 mins

INGREDIENTS

- 2 tablespoons psyllium husk powder
- ¾ cup coconut flour
- 1 teaspoon garlic powder
- ½ teaspoon salt
- ½ teaspoon baking soda
- 1 cup boiling water
- 1 teaspoon apple cider vinegar
- 3 eggs
- Toppings
- 3 tablespoons tomato sauce
- 1½ oz. Mozzarella cheese
- 1 tablespoon basil, freshly chopped

DIRECTIONS

1. Preheat the oven to 350 degrees F and grease a baking sheet.
2. Mix coconut flour, salt, psyllium husk powder, and garlic powder until fully combined.
3. Add eggs, apple cider vinegar, and baking soda and knead with boiling water.
4. Place the dough out on a baking sheet and top with the toppings.

5. Transfer in the oven and bake for about 20 minutes.
6. Dish out and serve warm.

NUTRITION: Calories: 173 Carbs: 16.8g Fats: 7.4g Proteins: 10.4g Sodium: 622mg Sugar: 0.9g

415. **Mini Pizza Crusts**

Servings: 4

Preparation time: 20 mins

INGREDIENTS

- 1 cup coconut flour, sifted
- 8 large eggs, 5 whole eggs and 3 egg whites
- ½ teaspoon baking powder
- Italian spices, to taste
- Salt and black pepper, to taste
- For the pizza sauce
- 2 garlic cloves, crushed
- 1 teaspoon dried basil
- ½ cup tomato sauce
- ¼ teaspoon sea salt

DIRECTIONS

- Preheat the oven to 350 degrees F and grease a baking tray.
- Whisk together eggs and egg whites in a large bowl and stir in the coconut flour, baking powder, Italian spices, salt, and black pepper.
- Make small dough balls from this mixture and press on the baking tray.
- Transfer in the oven and bake for about 20 minutes.
- Allow pizza bases to cool and keep aside.

- Combine all ingredients for the pizza sauce together and sit at room temperature for half an hour.
- Spread this pizza sauce over the pizza crusts and serve.

NUTRITION: Calories: 170 Carbs: 5.7g Fats: 10.5g Proteins: 13.6g Sodium: 461mg Sugar: 2.3g

416. **Keto Pepperoni Pizza**

Servings: 4

Preparation time: 40 mins

INGREDIENTS

- Crust
- 6 oz. mozzarella cheese, shredded
- 4 eggs
- Topping
- 1 teaspoon dried oregano
- 1½ oz. pepperoni
- 3 tablespoons tomato paste
- 5 oz. mozzarella cheese, shredded
- Olives

DIRECTIONS :

- Preheat the oven to 400 degrees F and grease a baking sheet.
- Whisk together eggs and cheese in a bowl and spread on a baking sheet.
- Transfer in the oven and bake for about 15 minutes until golden.
- Remove from the oven and allow it to cool.
- Increase the oven temperature to 450 degrees F.
- Spread the tomato paste on the crust and top with oregano, pepperoni, cheese, and olives on top.

- Bake for another 10 minutes and serve hot.

NUTRITION: Calories: 356 Carbs: 6.1g Fats: 23.8g Proteins: 30.6g Sodium: 790mg Sugar: 1.8g

417. Thin Crust Low Carb Pizza

Servings: 6

Preparation time: 25 mins

INGREDIENTS

- 2 tablespoons tomato sauce
- 1/8 teaspoon black pepper
- 1/8 teaspoon chili flakes
- 1 piece low-carb pita bread
- 2 ounces low-moisture mozzarella cheese
- 1/8 teaspoon garlic powder

Toppings:

- Bacon, roasted red peppers, spinach, olives, pesto, artichokes, salami, pepperoni, roast beef, prosciutto, avocado, ham, chili paste, Sriracha

DIRECTIONS

1. Preheat the oven to 450 degrees F and grease a baking dish.
2. Mix together tomato sauce, black pepper, chili flakes, and garlic powder in a bowl and keep aside.
3. Place the low-carb pita bread in the oven and bake for about 2 minutes.
4. Remove from oven and spread the tomato sauce on it.
5. Add mozzarella cheese and top with your favorite toppings.

6. Bake again for 3 minutes and dish out.

NUTRITION: Calories: 254 Carbs: 12.9g Fats: 16g Proteins: 19.3g Sodium: 255mg Sugar: 2.8g

418. BBQ Chicken Pizza

Servings: 4

Preparation time: 30 mins

INGREDIENTS

- Dairy Free Pizza Crust
- 6 tablespoons Parmesan cheese
- 6 large eggs
- 3 tablespoons psyllium husk powder
- Salt and black pepper, to taste
- 1½ teaspoons Italian seasoning
- Toppings
- 6 oz. rotisserie chicken, shredded
- 4 oz. cheddar cheese
- 1 tablespoon mayonnaise
- 4 tablespoons tomato sauce
- 4 tablespoons BBQ sauce

DIRECTIONS

1. Preheat the oven to 400 degrees F and grease a baking dish.
2. Place all Pizza Crust ingredients in an immersion blender and blend until smooth.
3. Spread dough mixture onto the baking dish and transfer in the oven.
4. Bake for about 10 minutes and top with favorite toppings.
5. Bake for about 3 minutes and dish out.

NUTRITION: Calories: 356 Carbs: 2.9g Fats: 24.5g Proteins: 24.5g Sodium: 396mg Sugar: 0.6g

419. <u>**Buffalo Chicken Crust Pizza**</u>

Servings: 6

Preparation time: 25 mins

INGREDIENTS

- 1 cup whole milk mozzarella, shredded
- 1 teaspoon dried oregano
- 2 tablespoons butter
- 1 pound chicken thighs, boneless and skinless
- 1 large egg
- ¼ teaspoon black pepper
- ¼ teaspoon salt
- 1 stalk celery
- 3 tablespoons Franks Red Hot Original
- 1 stalk green onion
- 1 tablespoon sour cream
- 1 ounce bleu cheese, crumbled

DIRECTIONS

1. Preheat the oven to 400 degrees F and grease a baking dish.
2. Process chicken thighs in a food processor until smooth.
3. Transfer to a large bowl and add egg, ½ cup of shredded mozzarella, oregano, black pepper, and salt to form a dough.
4. Spread the chicken dough in the baking dish and transfer in the oven
5. Bake for about 25 minutes and keep aside.
6. Meanwhile, heat butter and add celery, and cook for about 4 minutes.
7. Mix Franks Red Hot Original with the sour cream in a small bowl.

8. Spread the sauce mixture over the crust, layer with the cooked celery and remaining ½ cup of mozzarella and the bleu cheese.
9. Bake for another 10 minutes, until the cheese is melted

NUTRITION: Calories: 172 Carbs: 1g Fats: 12.9g Proteins: 13.8g Sodium: 172mg Sugar: 0.2g

420. <u>**Fresh Bell Pepper Basil Pizza**</u>

Servings: 3

Preparation time: 25 mins

INGREDIENTS

- Pizza Base
- ½ cup almond flour
- 2 tablespoons cream cheese
- 1 teaspoon Italian seasoning
- ½ teaspoon black pepper
- 6 ounces mozzarella cheese
- 2 tablespoons psyllium husk
- 2 tablespoons fresh Parmesan cheese
- 1 large egg
- ½ teaspoon salt
- Toppings
- 4 ounces cheddar cheese, shredded
- ¼ cup Marinara sauce
- 2/3 medium bell pepper
- 1 medium vine tomato
- 3 tablespoons basil, fresh chopped

DIRECTIONS :

1. Preheat the oven to 400 degrees F and grease a baking dish.

2. Microwave mozzarella cheese for about 30 seconds and top with the remaining pizza crust.
3. Add the remaining pizza ingredients to the cheese and mix together.
4. Flatten the dough and transfer in the oven.
5. Bake for about 10 minutes and remove pizza from the oven.
6. Top the pizza with the toppings and bake for another 10 minutes.
7. Remove pizza from the oven and allow to cool.

NUTRITION: Calories: 411 Carbs: 6.4g Fats: 31.3g Proteins: 22.2g Sodium: 152mg Sugar: 2.8g

421. Keto Thai Chicken Flatbread Pizza

Servings: 12

Preparation time: 25 mins

INGREDIENTS

- Peanut Sauce
- 2 tablespoons rice wine vinegar
- 4 tablespoons reduced sugar ketchup
- 4 tablespoons pbfit
- 4 tablespoons soy sauce
- 4 tablespoons coconut oil
- ½ lime, juiced
- 1 teaspoon fish sauce
- Pizza Base
- ¾ cup almond flour
- 3 tablespoons cream cheese
- ½ teaspoon garlic powder
- 8 oz. mozzarella cheese
- 1 tablespoon psyllium husk powder
- 1 large egg
- ½ teaspoon onion powder
- ½ teaspoon ginger
- ½ teaspoon black pepper
- ½ teaspoon salt
- Toppings
- 3 oz. mung bean sprouts
- 2 medium green onions
- 2 tablespoons peanuts
- 2 chicken thighs
- 6 oz. mozzarella cheese
- 1½ oz. carrots, shredded

DIRECTIONS

1. Preheat oven to 400 degrees F and grease a baking tray.
2. Mix together all peanut sauce ingredients and set aside.
3. Microwave cream cheese and mozzarella cheese for the pizza base for 1 minute.
4. Add eggs, then mix together with all dry ingredients.
5. Arrange dough onto a baking tray and bake for about 15 minutes.
6. Flip pizza and top with sauce, chopped chicken, shredded carrots, and mozzarella.
7. Bake again for 10 minutes, or until cheese has melted.
8. Top with bean sprouts, spring onion, peanuts, and cilantro.

NUTRITION: Calories: 268 Carbs: 3.2g Fats: 21g Proteins: 15g Sodium: 94mg Sugar: 0.2g

422. Apple and Ham Flatbread Pizza

Servings: 8

Preparation time: 15 mins

INGREDIENTS

For the crust:

- ¾ cup almond flour
- ½ teaspoon sea salt
- 2 cups mozzarella cheese, shredded
- 2 tablespoons cream cheese
- 1/8 teaspoon dried thyme

For the topping:

- ½ small red onion, cut into thin slices
- 4 ounces low carbohydrate ham, cut into chunks
- Salt and black pepper, to taste
- 1 cup Mexican blend cheese, grated
- ¼ medium apple, sliced
- 1/8 teaspoon dried thyme

DIRECTIONS

1. Preheat the oven to 425 degrees F and grease a 12-inch pizza pan.
2. Boil water and steam cream cheese, mozzarella cheese, almond flour, thyme, and salt.
3. When the cheese melts enough, knead for a few minutes to thoroughly mix dough.
4. Make a ball out of the dough and arrange in the pizza pan.
5. Poke holes all over the dough with a fork and transfer in the oven.
6. Bake for about 8 minutes until golden brown and reset the oven setting to 350 degrees F.
7. Sprinkle ¼ cup of the Mexican blend cheese over the flatbread and top with onions, apples, and ham.
8. Cover with the remaining ¾ cup of the Mexican blend cheese and sprinkle with the thyme, salt, and black pepper.

9. Bake for about 7 minutes until cheese is melted and crust is golden brown.
10. Remove the flatbread from the oven and allow to cool before cutting.
11. Slice into desired pieces and serve.

NUTRITION: Calories: 179 Carbs: 5.3g Fats: 13.6g Proteins: 10.4g Sodium: 539mg Sugar: 2.1g

Air Fryer Breakfast Recipes

423. <u>Ham, Spinach & Egg in a Cup</u>

Servings: 8

Preparation time: 35 mins

INGREDIENTS

- 2 tablespoons olive oil
- 2 tablespoons unsalted butter, melted
- 2 pounds fresh baby spinach
- 8 eggs
- 8 teaspoons milk
- 14-ounce ham, sliced
- Salt and black pepper, to taste

DIRECTIONS

1. Preheat the Airfryer to 360 degrees F and grease 8 ramekins with butter.
2. Heat oil in a skillet on medium heat and add spinach.
3. Cook for about 3 minutes and drain the liquid completely from the spinach.
4. Divide the spinach into prepared ramekins and layer with ham slices.
5. Crack 1 egg over ham slices into each ramekin and drizzle evenly with milk.
6. Sprinkle with salt and black pepper and bake for about 20 minutes.

NUTRITION:Calories: 228 Carbs: 6.6g Fats: 15.6g Proteins: 17.2g Sodium: 821mg Sugar: 1.1g

424. Eggs with Sausage & Bacon

Servings: 2

Preparation time: 25 mins

INGREDIENTS

- 4 chicken sausages
- 4 bacon slices
- 2 eggs
- Salt and freshly ground black pepper, to taste

DIRECTIONS

1. Preheat the Airfryer to 330 degrees F and place sausages and bacon slices in an Airfryer basket.
2. Cook for about 10 minutes and lightly grease 2 ramekins.
3. Crack 1 egg in each prepared ramekin and season with salt and black pepper.
4. Cook for about 10 minutes and divide sausages and bacon slices in serving plates.

NUTRITION: Calories: 245 Carbs: 5.7g Fats: 15.8g Proteins: 17.8g Sodium: 480mg Sugar: 0.7g

425. Tropical Almond Pancakes

Servings: 8

Preparation time: 15 mins

INGREDIENTS

- 2 cups creamy milk
- 3½ cups almond flour
- 1 teaspoon baking soda
- ½ teaspoon salt
- 1 teaspoon allspice
- 2 tablespoons vanilla
- 1 teaspoon cinnamon
- 1 teaspoon baking powder
- ½ cup club soda

DIRECTIONS

1. Preheat the Air fryer at 290 degrees F and grease the cooking basket of the air fryer.
2. Whisk together salt, almond flour, baking soda, allspice and cinnamon in a large bowl.
3. Mix together the vanilla, baking powder and club soda and add to the flour mixture.
4. Stir the mixture thoroughly and pour the mixture into the cooking basket.
5. Cook for about 10 minutes and dish out in a serving platter.

NUTRITION:Calories: 324 Carbs: 12.8g Fats: 24.5g Proteins: 11.4g Sodium: 342mg Sugar: 1.6g

426. Bacon & Hot Dogs Omelet

Servings: 4

Preparation time: 15 mins

INGREDIENTS

- 4 hot dogs, chopped
- 8 eggs
- 2 bacon slices, chopped
- 4 small onions, chopped

DIRECTIONS

1. Preheat the Airfryer to 325 degrees F.
2. Crack the eggs in an Airfryer baking pan and beat well.
3. Stir in the remaining ingredients and cook for about 10 minutes until completely done.

NUTRITION: Calories: 298 Carbs: 9g Fats: 21.8g   Proteins: 16.9g   Sodium: 628mg Sugar: 5.1g

427. **Toasted Bagels**

Servings: 6

Preparation time: 10 mins

INGREDIENTS

- 6 teaspoons butter
- 3 bagels, halved

DIRECTIONS

1. Preheat the Airfryer to 375 degrees F and arrange the bagels into an Airfryer basket.
2. Cook for about 3 minutes and remove the bagels from Airfryer.
3. Spread butter evenly over bagels and cook for about 3 more minutes.

NUTRITION: Calories: 169   Carbs: 26.5g Fats: 4.7g Proteins: 5.3g Sodium: 262mg Sugar: 2.7g

428. **Eggless Spinach & Bacon Quiche**

Servings: 8

Preparation time: 20 mins

INGREDIENTS

- 1 cup fresh spinach, chopped
- 4 slices of bacon, cooked and chopped
- ½ cup mozzarella cheese, shredded
- 4 tablespoons milk
- 4 dashes Tabasco sauce
- 1 cup Parmesan cheese, shredded
- Salt and freshly ground black pepper, to taste

DIRECTIONS

1. Preheat the Airfryer to 325 degrees F and grease a baking dish.
2. Put all the ingredients in a bowl and mix well.
3. Transfer the mixture into prepared baking dish and cook for about 8 minutes.
4. Dish out and serve.

NUTRITION: Calories: 72   Carbs: 0.9g Fats: 5.2g Proteins: 5.5g Sodium: 271mg Sugar: 0.4g

429. **Ham Casserole**

Servings: 4

Preparation time: 25 mins

INGREDIENTS

- 4-ounce ham, sliced thinly
- 4 teaspoons unsalted butter, softened
- 8 large eggs, divided
- 4 tablespoons heavy cream
- ¼ teaspoon smoked paprika
- 4 teaspoons fresh chives, minced
- Salt and freshly ground black pepper, to taste

- 6 tablespoons Parmesan cheese, grated finely

DIRECTIONS

1. Preheat the Airfryer to 325 degrees F and spread butter in the pie pan.
2. Place ham slices in the bottom of the pie pan.
3. Whisk together 2 eggs, cream, salt and black pepper until smooth.
4. Place the egg mixture evenly over the ham slices and crack the remaining eggs on top.
5. Season with paprika, salt and black pepper.
6. Top evenly with chives and cheese and place the pie pan in an Airfryer.
7. Cook for about 12 minutes and serve with toasted bread slices.

NUTRITION: Calories: 410 Carbs: 3.9g Fats: 30.8g Proteins: 31.2g Sodium: 933mg Sugar: 0.8g

430. Sausage & Bacon with Beans

Servings: 12

Preparation time: 30 mins

INGREDIENTS

1. 12 medium sausages
2. 12 bacon slices
3. 8 eggs
4. 2 cans baked beans
5. 12 bread slices, toasted

DIRECTIONS

1. Preheat the Airfryer at 325 degrees F and place sausages and bacon in a fryer basket.

2. Cook for about 10 minutes and place the baked beans in a ramekin.
3. Place eggs in another ramekin and the Airfryer to 395 degrees F.
4. Cook for about 10 more minutes and divide the sausage mixture, beans and eggs in serving plates
5. Serve with bread slices.

NUTRITION: Calories: 276 Carbs: 14.1g Fats: 17g Proteins: 16.3g Sodium: 817mg Sugar: 0.6g

431. French Toasts

Servings: 4

Preparation time: 15 mins

INGREDIENTS

- ½ cup evaporated milk
- 4 eggs
- 6 tablespoons sugar
- ¼ teaspoon vanilla extract
- 8 bread slices
- 4 teaspoons olive oil

DIRECTIONS

1. Preheat the Airfryer to 395 degrees F and grease a pan.
2. Put all the ingredients in a large shallow dish except the bread slices.
3. Beat till well combined and dip each bread slice in egg mixture from both sides.
4. Arrange the bread slices in the prepared pan and cook for about 3 minutes per side.

NUTRITION: Calories: 261 Carbs: 30.6g Fats: 12g Proteins: 9.1g Sodium: 218mg Sugar: 22.3g

432. Veggie Hash

Servings: 8

Preparation time: 55 mins

INGREDIENTS

- 2 medium onions, chopped
- 2 teaspoons dried thyme, crushed
- 4 teaspoons butter
- 1 green bell pepper, seeded and chopped
- 3 pounds russet potatoes, peeled and cubed
- Salt and freshly ground black pepper, to taste
- 10 eggs

DIRECTIONS

1. Preheat the Airfryer to 395 degrees F and grease the Airfryer pan with butter.
2. Add bell peppers and onions and cook for about 5 minutes.
3. Add the herbs, potatoes, salt and black pepper and cook for about 30 minutes.
4. Heat a greased skillet on medium heat and add beaten eggs.
5. Cook for about 1 minute on each side and remove from the skillet.
6. Cut it into small pieces and add egg pieces into Airfryer pan.
7. Cook for about 5 more minutes and dish out.

NUTRITION: Calories: 229 Carbs: 31g Fats: 7.6g Proteins: 10.3g Sodium: 102mg Sugar: 4.3g

433. Parmesan Garlic Rolls

Servings: 4

Preparation time: 15 mins

INGREDIENTS

- 1 cup Parmesan cheese, grated
- 4 dinner rolls
- 4 tablespoons unsalted butter, melted
- 1 tablespoon garlic bread seasoning mix

DIRECTIONS

1. Preheat the Airfryer at 360 degrees F and cut the dinner rolls into cross style.
2. Stuff the slits evenly with the cheese and coat the tops of each roll with butter.
3. Sprinkle with the seasoning mix and cook for about 5 minutes until cheese is fully melted.

NUTRITION: Calories: 391 Carbs: 45g Fats: 18.6g Proteins: 11.7g Sodium: 608mg Sugar: 4.8g

434. Pickled Toasts

Servings: 4

Preparation time: 25 mins

INGREDIENTS

- 4 tablespoons unsalted butter, softened
- 8 bread slices, toasted
- 4 tablespoons Branston pickle
- ½ cup Parmesan cheese, grated

DIRECTIONS

1. Preheat the Airfryer to 385 degrees F and place the bread slice in a fryer basket.
2. Cook for about 5 minutes and spread butter evenly over bread slices.
3. Layer with Branston pickle and top evenly with cheese.
4. Cook for about 5 minutes until cheese is fully melted.

NUTRITION: Calories: 186 Carbs: 16.3g Fats: 12.9g Proteins: 2.6g Sodium: 397mg Sugar: 6.8g

435. **Potato Rosti**

Servings: 4

Preparation time: 15 mins

INGREDIENTS

- ½ pound russet potatoes, peeled and grated roughly
- Salt and freshly ground black pepper, to taste
- 3.5 ounces smoked salmon, cut into slices
- k1 teaspoon olive oil
- 1 tablespoon chives, chopped finely
- 2 tablespoons sour cream

DIRECTIONS

1. Preheat the Airfryer to 360 degrees F and grease a pizza pan with the olive oil.
2. Add chives, potatoes, salt and black pepper in a large bowl and mix until well combined.

3. Place the potato mixture into the prepared pizza pan and transfer the pizza pan in an Airfryer basket.
4. Cook for about 15 minutes and cut the potato rosti into wedges.
5. Top with the smoked salmon slices and sour cream and serve.

NUTRITION: Calories: 91 Carbs: 9.2g Fats: 3.6g Proteins: 5.7g Sodium: 503mg Sugar: 0.7g

436. **Pumpkin Pancakes**

Servings: 8

Preparation time: 20 mins

INGREDIENTS

- 2 squares puff pastry
- 6 tablespoons pumpkin filling
- 2 small eggs, beaten
- ¼ teaspoon cinnamon

DIRECTIONS

1. Preheat the Airfryer to 360 degrees F and roll out a square of puff pastry.
2. Layer it with pumpkin pie filling, leaving about ¼-inch space around the edges.
3. Cut it up into equal sized square pieces and cover the gaps with beaten egg.
4. Arrange the squares into a baking dish and cook for about 12 minutes.
5. Sprinkle some cinnamon and serve.

NUTRITION: Calories: 51 Carbs: 5g Fats: 2.5g Proteins: 2.4g Sodium: 48mg Sugar: 0.5g

437. <u>Simple Cheese Sandwiches</u>

Servings: 4

Preparation time: 10 mins

INGREDIENTS

- 8 American cheese slices
- 8 bread slices
- 8 teaspoons butter

DIRECTIONS

1. Preheat the Air fryer to 365 degrees F and arrange cheese slices between bread slices.
2. Spread butter over outer sides of sandwich and repeat with the remaining butter, slices and cheese.
3. Arrange the sandwiches in an Air fryer basket and cook for about 8 minutes, flipping once in the middle way.

NUTRITION: Calories: 254 Carbs: 12.4g Fats: 18.8g Proteins: 9.2g Sodium: 708mg Sugar: 3.9g

SNACKS

438. Light & Creamy Garlic Hummus

Preparation Time: 10 minutes

Cooking Time: 40 minutes

Servings: 12

INGREDIENTS

- 1 1/2 cups dry chickpeas, rinsed
- 2 1/2 tbsp fresh lemon juice
- 1 tbsp garlic, minced
- 1/2 cup tahini
- 6 cups of water
- Pepper
- Salt

DIRECTIONS

1. Add water and chickpeas into the instant pot.
2. Seal pot with a lid and select manual and set timer for 40 minutes.
3. Once done, allow to release pressure naturally. Remove lid.
4. Drain chickpeas well and reserved 1/2 cup chickpeas liquid.
5. Transfer chickpeas, reserved liquid, lemon juice, garlic, tahini, pepper, and salt into the food processor and process until smooth.
6. Serve and enjoy.

NUTRITION: Calories 152 Fat 6.9 g Carbohydrates 17.6 g Sugar 2.8 g Protein 6.6 g Cholesterol 0 mg

439. Perfect Queso

Preparation Time: 10 minutes

Cooking Time: 15 minutes

Servings: 16

INGREDIENTS

- 1 lb ground beef
- 32 oz Velveeta cheese, cut into cubes
- 10 oz can tomatoes, diced
- 1 1/2 tbsp taco seasoning
- 1 tsp chili powder
- 1 onion, diced
- Pepper
- Salt

DIRECTIONS

1. Set instant pot on sauté mode.
2. Add meat, onion, taco seasoning, chili powder, pepper, and salt into the pot and cook until meat is no longer pink.
3. Add tomatoes and stir well. Top with cheese and do not stir.
4. Seal pot with lid and cook on high for 4 minutes.
5. Once done, release pressure using quick release. Remove lid.
6. Stir everything well and serve.

NUTRITION: Calories 257 Fat 15.9 g Carbohydrates 10.2 g Sugar 4.9 g Protein 21 g Cholesterol 71 mg

440. Creamy Potato Spread

Preparation Time: 10 minutes

Cooking Time: 15 minutes

Servings: 6

INGREDIENTS

- 1 lb sweet potatoes, peeled and chopped
- 3/4 tbsp fresh chives, chopped
- 1/2 tsp paprika
- 1 tbsp garlic, minced
- 1 cup tomato puree
- Pepper
- Salt

DIRECTIONS

1. Add all ingredients except chives into the inner pot of instant pot and stir well.
2. Seal pot with lid and cook on high for 15 minutes.
3. Once done, allow to release pressure naturally for 10 minutes then release remaining using quick release. Remove lid.
4. Transfer instant pot sweet potato mixture into the food processor and process until smooth.
5. Garnish with chives and serve.

NUTRITION: Calories 108 Fat 0.3 g Carbohydrates 25.4 g Sugar 2.4 g Protein 2 g Cholesterol 0 mg

441. Cucumber Tomato Okra Salsa

Preparation Time: 10 minutes

Cooking Time: 15 minutes

Servings: 4

INGREDIENTS

- 1 lb tomatoes, chopped
- 1/4 tsp red pepper flakes
- 1/4 cup fresh lemon juice
- 1 cucumber, chopped
- 1 tbsp fresh oregano, chopped
- 1 tbsp fresh basil, chopped
- 1 tbsp olive oil
- 1 onion, chopped
- 1 tbsp garlic, chopped
- 1 1/2 cups okra, chopped
- Pepper
- Salt

DIRECTIONS

1. Add oil into the inner pot of instant pot and set the pot on sauté mode.
2. Add onion, garlic, pepper, and salt and sauté for 3 minutes.
3. Add remaining ingredients except for cucumber and stir well.
4. Seal pot with lid and cook on high for 12 minutes.
5. Once done, allow to release pressure naturally for 10 minutes then release remaining using quick release. Remove lid.
6. Once the salsa mixture is cool then add cucumber and mix well.
7. Serve and enjoy.

NUTRITION: Calories 99 Fat 4.2 g Carbohydrates 14.3 g Sugar 6.4 g Protein 2.9 g Cholesterol 0 mg

442. Parmesan Potatoes

Preparation Time: 10 minutes

Cooking Time: 6 minutes

Servings: 4

INGREDIENTS

- 2 lb potatoes, rinsed and cut into chunks
- 2 tbsp parmesan cheese, grated
- 2 tbsp olive oil
- 1/2 tsp parsley
- 1/2 tsp Italian seasoning
- 1 tsp garlic, minced
- 1 cup vegetable broth
- 1/2 tsp salt

DIRECTIONS

1. Add all ingredients except cheese into the instant pot and stir well.
2. Seal pot with lid and cook on high for 6 minutes.
3. Once done, release pressure using quick release. Remove lid.
4. Add parmesan cheese and stir until cheese is melted.
5. Serve and enjoy.

NUTRITION: Calories 237 Fat 8.3 g Carbohydrates 36.3 g Sugar 2.8 g Protein 5.9 g Cholesterol 2 mg

443. Creamy Artichoke Dip

Preparation Time: 10 minutes

Cooking Time: 5 minutes

Servings: 8

INGREDIENTS

- 28 oz can artichoke hearts, drain and quartered
- 1 1/2 cups parmesan cheese, shredded
- 1 cup sour cream
- 1 cup mayonnaise
- 3.5 oz can green chilies
- 1 cup of water
- Pepper
- Salt

DIRECTIONS

1. Add artichokes, water, and green chilis into the instant pot.
2. Seal pot with the lid and select manual and set timer for 1 minute.
3. Once done, release pressure using quick release. Remove lid. Drain excess water.
4. Set instant pot on sauté mode. Add remaining ingredients and stir well and cook until cheese is melted.
5. Serve and enjoy.

NUTRITION: Calories 262 Fat 7.6 g Carbohydrates 14.4 g Sugar 2.8 g Protein 8.4 g Cholesterol 32 mg

444. Homemade Salsa

Preparation Time: 10 minutes

Cooking Time: 5 minutes

Servings: 8

INGREDIENTS

- 12 oz grape tomatoes, halved
- 1/4 cup fresh cilantro, chopped
- 1 fresh lime juice
- 28 oz tomatoes, crushed
- 1 tbsp garlic, minced
- 1 green bell pepper, chopped
- 1 red bell pepper, chopped
- 2 onions, chopped
- 6 whole tomatoes
- Salt

DIRECTIONS

1. Add whole tomatoes into the instant pot and gently smash the tomatoes.
2. Add remaining ingredients except cilantro, lime juice, and salt and stir well.
3. Seal pot with lid and cook on high for 5 minutes.
4. Once done, allow to release pressure naturally for 10 minutes then release remaining using quick release. Remove lid.
5. Add cilantro, lime juice, and salt and stir well.
6. Serve and enjoy.

NUTRITION: Calories 146 Fat 1.2 g Carbohydrates 33.2 g Sugar 4 g Protein 6.9 g Cholesterol 0 mg

445. Delicious Eggplant Caponata

Preparation Time: 10 minutes

Cooking Time: 5 minutes

Servings: 8

INGREDIENTS

- 1 eggplant, cut into 1/2-inch chunks
- 1 lb tomatoes, diced
- 1/2 cup tomato puree
- 1/4 cup dates, chopped
- 2 tbsp vinegar
- 1/2 cup fresh parsley, chopped
- 2 celery stalks, chopped
- 1 small onion, chopped
- 2 zucchini, cut into 1/2-inch chunks
- Pepper
- Salt

DIRECTIONS

1. Add all ingredients into the inner pot of instant pot and stir well.
2. Seal pot with lid and cook on high for 5 minutes.
3. Once done, release pressure using quick release. Remove lid.
4. Stir well and serve.

NUTRITION: Calories 60 Fat 0.4 g Carbohydrates 14 g Sugar 8.8 g Protein 2.3 g Cholesterol 0.4 mg

446. Flavorful Roasted Baby Potatoes

Preparation Time: 10 minutes

Cooking Time: 10 minutes

Servings: 4

INGREDIENTS

- 2 lbs baby potatoes, clean and cut in half
- 1/2 cup vegetable stock
- 1 tsp paprika
- 3/4 tsp garlic powder
- 1 tsp onion powder
- 2 tsp Italian seasoning
- 1 tbsp olive oil
- Pepper
- Salt

DIRECTIONS

1. Add oil into the inner pot of instant pot and set the pot on sauté mode.
2. Add potatoes and sauté for 5 minutes. Add remaining ingredients and stir well.
3. Seal pot with lid and cook on high for 5 minutes.
4. Once done, release pressure using quick release. Remove lid.
5. Stir well and serve.

NUTRITION: Calories 175 Fat 4.5 g Carbohydrates 29.8 g Sugar 0.7 g Protein 6.1 g Cholesterol 2 mg

447. **Perfect Italian Potatoes**

Preparation Time: 10 minutes

Cooking Time: 7 minutes

Servings: 6

INGREDIENTS

- 2 lbs baby potatoes, clean and cut in half
- 3/4 cup vegetable broth
- 6 oz Italian dry dressing mix

DIRECTIONS

1. Add all ingredients into the inner pot of instant pot and stir well.
2. Seal pot with lid and cook on high for 7 minutes.
3. Once done, allow to release pressure naturally for 3 minutes then release remaining using quick release. Remove lid.
4. Stir well and serve.

NUTRITION: Calories 149 Fat 0.3 g Carbohydrates 41.6 g Sugar 11.4 g Protein 4.5 g Cholesterol 0 mg

448. **Garlic Pinto Bean Dip**

Preparation Time: 10 minutes

Cooking Time: 43 minutes

Servings: 6

INGREDIENTS

- 1 cup dry pinto beans, rinsed
- 1/2 tsp cumin
- 1/2 cup salsa
- 2 garlic cloves
- 2 chipotle peppers in adobo sauce
- 5 cups vegetable stock
- Pepper
- Salt

DIRECTIONS

1. Add beans, stock, garlic, and chipotle peppers into the instant pot.
2. Seal pot with lid and cook on high for 43 minutes.
3. Once done, release pressure using quick release. Remove lid.
4. Drain beans well and reserve 1/2 cup of stock.

5. Transfer beans, reserve stock, and remaining ingredients into the food processor and process until smooth.
6. Serve and enjoy.

NUTRITION: Calories 129 Fat 0.9 g Carbohydrates 23 g Sugar 1.9 g Protein 8 g Cholesterol 2 mg

449. <u>Creamy Eggplant Dip</u>

Preparation Time: 10 minutes

Cooking Time: 20 minutes

Servings: 4

INGREDIENTS

- 1 eggplant
- 1/2 tsp paprika
- 1 tbsp olive oil
- 1 tbsp fresh lime juice
- 2 tbsp tahini
- 1 garlic clove
- 1 cup of water
- Pepper
- Salt

DIRECTIONS

1. Add water and eggplant into the instant pot.
2. Seal pot with the lid and select manual and set timer for 20 minutes.
3. Once done, release pressure using quick release. Remove lid.
4. Drain eggplant and let it cool.
5. Once the eggplant is cool then remove eggplant skin and transfer eggplant flesh into the food processor.
6. Add remaining ingredients into the food processor and process until smooth.

7. Serve and enjoy.

NUTRITION: Calories 108 Fat 7.8 g Carbohydrates 9.7 g Sugar 3.7 g Protein 2.5 g Cholesterol 0 mg

450. <u>Jalapeno Chickpea Hummus</u>

Preparation Time: 10 minutes

Cooking Time: 25 minutes

Servings: 4

INGREDIENTS

- 1 cup dry chickpeas, soaked overnight and drained
- 1 tsp ground cumin
- 1/4 cup jalapenos, diced
- 1/2 cup fresh cilantro
- 1 tbsp tahini
- 1/2 cup olive oil
- Pepper
- Salt

DIRECTIONS

1. Add chickpeas into the instant pot and cover with vegetable stock.
2. Seal pot with lid and cook on high for 25 minutes.
3. Once done, allow to release pressure naturally. Remove lid.
4. Drain chickpeas well and transfer into the food processor along with remaining ingredients and process until smooth.
5. Serve and enjoy.

NUTRITION: Calories 425 Fat 30.4 g Carbohydrates 31.8 g Sugar 5.6 g Protein 10.5 g Cholesterol 0 mg

451. <u>Tasty Black Bean Dip</u>

Preparation Time: 10 minutes

Cooking Time: 18 minutes

Servings: 6

INGREDIENTS

- 2 cups dry black beans, soaked overnight and drained
- 1 1/2 cups cheese, shredded
- 1 tsp dried oregano
- 1 1/2 tsp chili powder
- 2 cups tomatoes, chopped
- 2 tbsp olive oil
- 1 1/2 tbsp garlic, minced
- 1 medium onion, sliced
- 4 cups vegetable stock
- Pepper
- Salt

DIRECTIONS

1. Add all ingredients except cheese into the instant pot.
2. Seal pot with lid and cook on high for 18 minutes.
3. Once done, allow to release pressure naturally. Remove lid. Drain excess water.
4. Add cheese and stir until cheese is melted.
5. Blend bean mixture using an immersion blender until smooth.
6. Serve and enjoy.

NUTRITION: Calories 402 Fat 15.3 g Carbohydrates 46.6 g Sugar 4.4 g Protein 22.2 g Cholesterol 30 mg

452. <u>Healthy Kidney Bean Dip</u>

Preparation Time: 10 minutes

Cooking Time: 10 minutes

Servings: 6

INGREDIENTS

- 1 cup dry white kidney beans, soaked overnight and drained
- 1 tbsp fresh lemon juice
- 2 tbsp water
- 1/2 cup coconut yogurt
- 1 roasted garlic clove
- 1 tbsp olive oil
- 1/4 tsp cayenne
- 1 tsp dried parsley
- Pepper
- Salt

DIRECTIONS

1. Add soaked beans and 1 3/4 cups of water into the instant pot.
2. Seal pot with lid and cook on high for 10 minutes.
3. Once done, allow to release pressure naturally. Remove lid.
4. Drain beans well and transfer them into the food processor.
5. Add remaining ingredients into the food processor and process until smooth.
6. Serve and enjoy.

NUTRITION: Calories 136 Fat 3.2 g Carbohydrates 20 g Sugar 2.1 g Protein 7.7 g Cholesterol 0 mg

453. <u>Creamy Pepper Spread</u>

Preparation Time: 10 minutes

Cooking Time: 15 minutes

Servings: 4

INGREDIENTS

- 1 lb red bell peppers, chopped and remove seeds
- 1 1/2 tbsp fresh basil
- 1 tbsp olive oil
- 1 tbsp fresh lime juice
- 1 tsp garlic, minced
- Pepper
- Salt

DIRECTIONS

1. Add all ingredients into the inner pot of instant pot and stir well.
2. Seal pot with lid and cook on high for 15 minutes.
3. Once done, allow to release pressure naturally for 10 minutes then release remaining using quick release. Remove lid.
4. Transfer bell pepper mixture into the food processor and process until smooth.
5. Serve and enjoy.

NUTRITION: Calories 41 Fat 3.6 g Carbohydrates 3.5 g Sugar 1.7 g Protein 0.4 g Cholesterol 0 mg

454. <u>Healthy Spinach Dip</u>

Preparation Time: 10 minutes

Cooking Time: 8 minutes

Servings: 4

INGREDIENTS

- 14 oz spinach
- 2 tbsp fresh lime juice
- 1 tbsp garlic, minced
- 2 tbsp olive oil
- 2 tbsp coconut cream
- Pepper
- Salt

DIRECTIONS

1. Add all ingredients except coconut cream into the instant pot and stir well.
2. Seal pot with lid and cook on low pressure for 8 minutes.
3. Once done, allow to release pressure naturally for 5 minutes then release remaining using quick release. Remove lid.
4. Add coconut cream and stir well and blend spinach mixture using a blender until smooth.
5. Serve and enjoy.

NUTRITION: Calories 109 Fat 9.2 g Carbohydrates 6.6 g Sugar 1.1 g Protein 3.2 g Cholesterol 0 mg

<u>Kidney Bean Spread</u>

Preparation Time: 10 minutes

Cooking Time: 18 minutes

Servings: 4

INGREDIENTS

- 1 lb dry kidney beans, soaked overnight and drained
- 1 tsp garlic, minced

- 2 tbsp olive oil
- 1 tbsp fresh lemon juice
- 1 tbsp paprika
- 4 cups vegetable stock
- 1/2 cup onion, chopped
- Pepper
- Salt

DIRECTIONS

1. Add beans and stock into the instant pot.
2. Seal pot with lid and cook on high for 18 minutes.
3. Once done, allow to release pressure naturally. Remove lid.
4. Drain beans well and reserve 1/2 cup stock.
5. Transfer beans, reserve stock, and remaining ingredients into the food processor and process until smooth.
6. Serve and enjoy.

NUTRITION: Calories 461 Fat 8.6 g Carbohydrates 73 g Sugar 4 g Protein 26.4 g Cholesterol 0 mg

455. Tomato Cucumber Salsa

Preparation Time: 10 minutes

Cooking Time: 5 minutes

Servings: 4

INGREDIENTS

- 1 cucumber, chopped
- 1 1/2 lbs grape tomatoes, chopped
- 1 tbsp fresh chives, chopped
- 1 tbsp fresh parsley, chopped
- 1 tbsp fresh basil, chopped
- 2 onion, chopped
- 1/4 cup vinegar

- 2 tbsp olive oil
- 1/4 cup vegetable stock
- 2 chili peppers, chopped
- Pepper
- Salt

DIRECTIONS

1. Add tomatoes, stock, and chili peppers into the instant pot and stir well.
2. Seal pot with lid and cook on low pressure for 5 minutes.
3. Once done, allow to release pressure naturally for 5 minutes then release remaining using quick release. Remove lid.
4. Transfer tomato mixture into the mixing bowl.
5. Add remaining ingredients into the bowl and mix well.
6. Serve and enjoy.

NUTRITION: Calories 129 Fat 7.5 g Carbohydrates 15 g Sugar 8.3 g Protein 2.7 g Cholesterol 0 mg

456. Spicy Berry Dip

Preparation Time: 10 minutes

Cooking Time: 15 minutes

Servings: 4

INGREDIENTS

- 10 oz cranberries
- 1/4 cup fresh orange juice
- 3/4 tsp paprika
- 1/2 tsp chili powder
- 1 tsp lemon zest
- 1 tbsp lemon juice

DIRECTIONS

1. Add all ingredients into the inner pot of instant pot and stir well.
2. Seal pot with lid and cook on high for 15 minutes.
3. Once done, allow to release pressure naturally for 5 minutes then release remaining using quick release. Remove lid.
4. Blend cranberry mixture using a blender until getting the desired consistency.
5. Serve and enjoy.

NUTRITION: Calories 49 Fat 0.2 g Carbohydrates 8.6 g Sugar 4.1 g Protein 0.3 g Cholesterol 0 mg

457. <u>Rosemary Cauliflower Dip</u>

Preparation Time: 10 minutes

Cooking Time: 15 minutes

Servings: 4

INGREDIENTS

- 1 lb cauliflower florets
- 1 tbsp fresh parsley, chopped
- 1/2 cup heavy cream
- 1/2 cup vegetable stock
- 1 tbsp garlic, minced
- 1 tbsp rosemary, chopped
- 1 tbsp olive oil
- 1 onion, chopped
- Pepper
- Salt

DIRECTIONS

1. Add oil into the inner pot of instant pot and set the pot on sauté mode.

2. Add onion and sauté for 5 minutes.
3. Add remaining ingredients except for parsley and heavy cream and stir well.
4. Seal pot with lid and cook on high for 10 minutes.
5. Once done, allow to release pressure naturally for 10 minutes then release remaining using quick release. Remove lid.
6. Add cream and stir well. Blend cauliflower mixture using immersion blender until smooth.
7. Garnish with parsley and serve.

NUTRITION: Calories 128 Fat 9.4 g Carbohydrates 10.4 g Sugar 4 g Protein 3.1 g Cholesterol 21 mg

458. <u>Tomato Olive Salsa</u>

Preparation Time: 10 minutes

Cooking Time: 5 minutes

Servings: 4

INGREDIENTS

- 2 cups olives, pitted and chopped
- 1/4 cup fresh parsley, chopped
- 1/4 cup fresh basil, chopped
- 2 tbsp green onion, chopped
- 1 cup grape tomatoes, halved
- 1 tbsp olive oil
- 1 tbsp vinegar
- Pepper
- Salt

DIRECTIONS

1. Add all ingredients into the inner pot of instant pot and stir well.
2. Seal pot with lid and cook on high for 5 minutes.

3. Once done, allow to release pressure naturally for 5 minutes then release remaining using quick release. Remove lid.
4. Stir well and serve.

NUTRITION: Calories 119 Fat 10.8 g Carbohydrates 6.5 g Sugar 1.3 g Protein 1.2 g Cholesterol 0 mg

459. Easy Tomato Dip

Preparation Time: 10 minutes

Cooking Time: 13 minutes

Servings: 4

INGREDIENTS

- 2 cups tomato puree
- 1/2 tsp ground cumin
- 1 tsp garlic, minced
- 1/4 cup vinegar
- 1 onion, chopped
- 1 tbsp olive oil
- Pepper
- Salt

DIRECTIONS

1. Add oil into the inner pot of instant pot and set the pot on sauté mode.
2. Add onion and sauté for 3 minutes.
3. Add remaining ingredients and stir well.
4. Seal pot with lid and cook on high for 10 minutes.
5. Once done, allow to release pressure naturally for 10 minutes then release remaining using quick release. Remove lid.
6. Blend tomato mixture using an immersion blender until smooth.

7. Serve and enjoy.

NUTRITION: Calories 94 Fat 3.9 g Carbohydrates 14.3 g Sugar 7.3 g Protein 2.5 g Cholesterol 0 mg

460. Balsamic Bell Pepper Salsa

Preparation Time: 10 minutes

Cooking Time: 6 minutes

Servings: 2

INGREDIENTS

- 2 red bell peppers, chopped and seeds removed
- 1 cup grape tomatoes, halved
- 1/2 tbsp cayenne
- 1 tbsp balsamic vinegar
- 2 cup vegetable broth
- 1/2 cup sour cream
- 1/2 tsp garlic powder
- 1/2 onion, chopped
- Salt

DIRECTIONS

1. Add all ingredients except cream into the instant pot and stir well.
2. Seal pot with lid and cook on high for 6 minutes.
3. Once done, release pressure using quick release. Remove lid.
4. Add sour cream and stir well.
5. Blend the salsa mixture using an immersion blender until smooth.
6. Serve and enjoy.

NUTRITION: Calories 235 Fat 14.2 g Carbohydrates 19.8 g Sugar 10.7 g Protein 9.2 g Cholesterol 25 mg

461. Spicy Chicken Dip

Preparation Time: 10 minutes

Cooking Time: 15 minutes

Servings: 10

INGREDIENTS

- 1 lb chicken breast, skinless and boneless
- 1/2 cup sour cream
- 8 oz cheddar cheese, shredded
- 1/2 cup chicken stock
- 2 jalapeno pepper, sliced
- 8 oz cream cheese
- Pepper
- Salt

DIRECTIONS

1. Add chicken, stock, jalapenos, and cream cheese into the instant pot.
2. Seal pot with lid and cook on high for 12 minutes.
3. Once done, release pressure using quick release. Remove lid.
4. Shred chicken using a fork.
5. Set pot on sauté mode. Add remaining ingredients and stir well and cook until cheese is melted.
6. Serve and enjoy.

NUTRITION: Calories 248 Fat 19 g Carbohydrates 1.6 g Sugar 0.3 g Protein 17.4 g Cholesterol 83 mg

462. Slow Cooked Cheesy Artichoke Dip

Preparation Time: 10 minutes

Cooking Time: 60 minutes

Servings: 6

INGREDIENTS

- 10 oz can artichoke hearts, drained and chopped
- 4 cups spinach, chopped
- 8 oz cream cheese
- 3 tbsp sour cream
- 1/4 cup mayonnaise
- 3/4 cup mozzarella cheese, shredded
- 1/4 cup parmesan cheese, grated
- 3 garlic cloves, minced
- 1/2 tsp dried parsley
- Pepper
- Salt

DIRECTIONS

1. Add all ingredients into the inner pot of instant pot and stir well.
2. Seal the pot with the lid and select slow cook mode and set the timer for 60 minutes. Stir once while cooking.
3. Serve and enjoy.

NUTRITION: Calories 226 Fat 19.3 g Carbohydrates 7.5 g Sugar 1.2 g Protein 6.8 g Cholesterol 51 mg

463. Olive Eggplant Spread

Preparation Time: 10 minutes

Cooking Time: 8 minutes

Servings: 12

INGREDIENTS

- 1 3/4 lbs eggplant, chopped
- 1/2 tbsp dried oregano
- 1/4 cup olives, pitted and chopped
- 1 tbsp tahini

- 1/4 cup fresh lime juice
- 1/2 cup water
- 2 garlic cloves
- 1/4 cup olive oil
- Salt

DIRECTIONS

1. Add oil into the inner pot of instant pot and set the pot on sauté mode.
2. Add eggplant and cook for 3-5 minutes. Turn off sauté mode.
3. Add water and salt and stir well.
4. Seal pot with lid and cook on high for 3 minutes.
5. Once done, release pressure using quick release. Remove lid.
6. Drain eggplant well and transfer into the food processor.
7. Add remaining ingredients into the food processor and process until smooth.
8. Serve and enjoy.

NUTRITION: Calories 65 Fat 5.3 g Carbohydrates 4.7 g Sugar 2 g Protein 0.9 g Cholesterol 0 mg

464. Pepper Tomato Eggplant Spread

Preparation Time: 10 minutes

Cooking Time: 10 minutes

Servings: 3

INGREDIENTS

- 2 cups eggplant, chopped
- 1/4 cup vegetable broth
- 2 tbsp tomato paste
- 1/4 cup sun-dried tomatoes, minced
- 1 cup bell pepper, chopped
- 1 tsp garlic, minced
- 1 cup onion, chopped
- 3 tbsp olive oil
- Salt

DIRECTIONS

1. Add oil into the inner pot of instant pot and set the pot on sauté mode.
2. Add onion and sauté for 3 minutes.
3. Add eggplant, bell pepper, and garlic and sauté for 2 minutes.
4. Add remaining ingredients and stir well.
5. Seal pot with lid and cook on high for 5 minutes.
6. Once done, release pressure using quick release. Remove lid.
7. Lightly mash the eggplant mixture using a potato masher.
8. Stir well and serve.

NUTRITION: Calories 178 Fat 14.4 g Carbohydrates 12.8 g Sugar 7 g Protein 2.4 g Cholesterol 0 mg

DESSERTS & FRUIT

465. Vanilla Apple Compote

Preparation Time: 10 minutes

Cooking Time: 15 minutes

Servings: 6

INGREDIENTS

- 3 cups apples, cored and cubed
- 1 tsp vanilla
- 3/4 cup coconut sugar
- 1 cup of water
- 2 tbsp fresh lime juice

DIRECTIONS

1. Add all ingredients into the inner pot of instant pot and stir well.
2. Seal pot with lid and cook on high for 15 minutes.
3. Once done, allow to release pressure naturally for 10 minutes then release remaining using quick release. Remove lid.
4. Stir and serve.

NUTRITION: Calories 76 Fat 0.2 g Carbohydrates 19.1 g Sugar 11.9 g Protein 0.5 g Cholesterol 0 mg

466. Apple Dates Mix

Preparation Time: 10 minutes

Cooking Time: 15 minutes

Servings: 4

INGREDIENTS

- 4 apples, cored and cut into chunks
- 1 tsp vanilla
- 1 tsp cinnamon
- 1/2 cup dates, pitted
- 1 1/2 cups apple juice

DIRECTIONS

1. Add all ingredients into the inner pot of instant pot and stir well.
2. Seal pot with lid and cook on high for 15 minutes.
3. Once done, allow to release pressure naturally for 10 minutes then release remaining using quick release. Remove lid.
4. Stir and serve.

NUTRITION: Calories 226 Fat 0.6 g Carbohydrates 58.6 g Sugar 46.4 g Protein 1.3 g Cholesterol 0 mg

467. Choco Rice Pudding

Preparation Time: 10 minutes

Cooking Time: 20 minutes

Servings: 4

INGREDIENTS

- 1 1/4 cup rice
- 1/4 cup dark chocolate, chopped
- 1 tsp vanilla
- 1/3 cup coconut butter
- 1 tsp liquid stevia
- 2 1/2 cups almond milk

DIRECTIONS

1. Add all ingredients into the inner pot of instant pot and stir well.
2. Seal pot with lid and cook on high for 20 minutes.
3. Once done, allow to release pressure naturally. Remove lid.
4. Stir well and serve.

NUTRITION: Calories 632 Fat 39.9 g Carbohydrates 63.5 g Sugar 12.5 g Protein 8.6 g Cholesterol 2 mg

468. Grapes Stew

Preparation Time: 10 minutes

Cooking Time: 15 minutes

Servings: 4

INGREDIENTS

- 1 cup grapes, halved
- 1 tsp vanilla
- 1 tbsp fresh lemon juice
- 1 tbsp honey
- 2 cups rhubarb, chopped
- 2 cups of water

DIRECTIONS

1. Add all ingredients into the inner pot of instant pot and stir well.
2. Seal pot with lid and cook on high for 15 minutes.
3. Once done, allow to release pressure naturally for 10 minutes then release remaining using quick release. Remove lid.
4. Stir and serve.

NUTRITION: Calories 48 Fat 0.2 g Carbohydrates 11.3 g Sugar 8.9 g Protein 0.7 g Cholesterol 0 mg

469. Chocolate Rice

Preparation Time: 10 minutes

Cooking Time: 20 minutes

Servings: 4

INGREDIENTS

- 1 cup of rice
- 1 tbsp cocoa powder
- 2 tbsp maple syrup
- 2 cups almond milk

DIRECTIONS

1. Add all ingredients into the inner pot of instant pot and stir well.
2. Seal pot with lid and cook on high for 20 minutes.
3. Once done, allow to release pressure naturally for 10 minutes then release remaining using quick release. Remove lid.
4. Stir and serve.

NUTRITION: Calories 474 Fat 29.1 g Carbohydrates 51.1 g Sugar 10 g Protein 6.3 g Cholesterol 0 mg

470. Raisins Cinnamon Peaches

Preparation Time: 10 minutes

Cooking Time: 15 minutes

Servings: 4

INGREDIENTS

- 4 peaches, cored and cut into chunks
- 1 tsp vanilla
- 1 tsp cinnamon
- 1/2 cup raisins
- 1 cup of water

DIRECTIONS

1. Add all ingredients into the inner pot of instant pot and stir well.
2. Seal pot with lid and cook on high for 15 minutes.
3. Once done, allow to release pressure naturally for 10 minutes then release remaining using quick release. Remove lid.
4. Stir and serve.

NUTRITION: Calories 118 Fat 0.5 g Carbohydrates 29 g Sugar 24.9 g Protein 2 g Cholesterol 0 mg

471. **Lemon Pear Compote**

Preparation Time: 10 minutes

Cooking Time: 15 minutes

Servings: 6

INGREDIENTS

- 3 cups pears, cored and cut into chunks
- 1 tsp vanilla
- 1 tsp liquid stevia
- 1 tbsp lemon zest, grated
- 2 tbsp lemon juice

DIRECTIONS

1. Add all ingredients into the inner pot of instant pot and stir well.
2. Seal pot with lid and cook on high for 15 minutes.
3. Once done, allow to release pressure naturally for 10 minutes then release remaining using quick release. Remove lid.
4. Stir and serve.

NUTRITION: Calories 50 Fat 0.2 g Carbohydrates 12.7 g Sugar 8.1 g Protein 0.4 g Cholesterol 0 mg

472. **Strawberry Stew**

Preparation Time: 10 minutes

Cooking Time: 15 minutes

Servings: 4

INGREDIENTS

- 12 oz fresh strawberries, sliced
- 1 tsp vanilla
- 1 1/2 cups water
- 1 tsp liquid stevia
- 2 tbsp lime juice

DIRECTIONS

1. Add all ingredients into the inner pot of instant pot and stir well.
2. Seal pot with lid and cook on high for 15 minutes.
3. Once done, allow to release pressure naturally for 10 minutes then release remaining using quick release. Remove lid.
4. Stir and serve.

NUTRITION: Calories 36 Fat 0.3 g Carbohydrates 8.5 g Sugar 4.7 g Protein 0.7 g Cholesterol 0 mg

473. Walnut Apple Pear Mix

Preparation Time: 10 minutes

Cooking Time: 10 minutes

Servings: 4

INGREDIENTS

- 2 apples, cored and cut into wedges
- 1/2 tsp vanilla
- 1 cup apple juice
- 2 tbsp walnuts, chopped
- 2 apples, cored and cut into wedges

DIRECTIONS

1. Add all ingredients into the inner pot of instant pot and stir well.
2. Seal pot with lid and cook on high for 10 minutes.
3. Once done, allow to release pressure naturally for 10 minutes then release remaining using quick release. Remove lid.
4. Serve and enjoy.

NUTRITION: Calories 132 Fat 2.6 g Carbohydrates 28.3 g Sugar 21.9 g Protein 1.3 g Cholesterol 0 mg

474. Cinnamon Pear Jam

Preparation Time: 10 minutes

Cooking Time: 4 minutes

Servings: 12

INGREDIENTS

- 8 pears, cored and cut into quarters
- 1 tsp cinnamon
- 1/4 cup apple juice
- 2 apples, peeled, cored and diced

DIRECTIONS

1. Add all ingredients into the inner pot of instant pot and stir well.
2. Seal pot with lid and cook on high for 4 minutes.
3. Once done, allow to release pressure naturally. Remove lid.
4. Blend pear apple mixture using an immersion blender until smooth.
5. Serve and enjoy.

NUTRITION: Calories 103 Fat 0.3 g Carbohydrates 27.1 g Sugar 18 g Protein 0.6 g Cholesterol 0 mg

475. Delicious Apple Pear Cobbler

Preparation Time: 10 minutes

Cooking Time: 12 minutes

Servings: 4

INGREDIENTS

- 3 apples, cored and cut into chunks
- 1 cup steel-cut oats
- 2 pears, cored and cut into chunks
- 1/4 cup maple syrup
- 1 1/2 cups water
- 1 tsp cinnamon

DIRECTIONS

1. Spray instant pot from inside with cooking spray.
2. Add all ingredients into the inner pot of instant pot and stir well.
3. Seal pot with lid and cook on high for 12 minutes.
4. Once done, release pressure using quick release. Remove lid.
5. Sere and enjoy.

NUTRITION: Calories 278 Fat 1.8 g Carbohydrates 66.5 g Sugar 39.5 g Protein 3.5 g Cholesterol 0 mg

476. Coconut Rice Pudding

Preparation Time: 10 minutes

Cooking Time: 3 minutes

Servings: 4

INGREDIENTS

- 1/2 cup rice
- 1/4 cup shredded coconut
- 3 tbsp swerve
- 1 1/2 cups water
- 14 oz can coconut milk
- Pinch of salt

DIRECTIONS

1. Spray instant pot from inside with cooking spray.
2. Add all ingredients into the inner pot of instant pot and stir well.
3. Seal pot with lid and cook on high for 3 minutes.
4. Once done, allow to release pressure naturally for 10 minutes then release remaining using quick release. Remove lid.
5. Serve and enjoy.

NUTRITION: Calories 298 Fat 23 g Carbohydrates 33.3 gSugar 11.6 g Protein 3.8 g Cholesterol 0 mg

477. Pear Sauce

Preparation Time: 10 minutes

Cooking Time: 15 minutes

Servings: 6

INGREDIENTS

- 10 pears, sliced
- 1 cup apple juice
- 1 1/2 tsp cinnamon
- 1/4 tsp nutmeg

DIRECTIONS

1. Add all ingredients into the instant pot and stir well.
2. Seal pot with lid and cook on high for 15 minutes.
3. Once done, allow to release pressure naturally for 10 minutes then release remaining using quick release. Remove lid.
4. Blend the pear mixture using an immersion blender until smooth.
5. Serve and enjoy.

NUTRITION: Calories 222 Fat 0.6 g Carbohydrates 58.2 g Sugar 38 g Protein 1.3 g Cholesterol 0 mg

478. Sweet Peach Jam

Preparation Time: 10 minutes

Cooking Time: 16 minutes

Servings: 20

INGREDIENTS

- 1 1/2 lb fresh peaches, pitted and chopped
- 1/2 tbsp vanilla
- 1/4 cup maple syrup

DIRECTIONS

1. Add all ingredients into the instant pot and stir well.
2. Seal pot with lid and cook on high for 1 minute.
3. Once done, allow to release pressure naturally. Remove lid.
4. Set pot on sauté mode and cook for 15 minutes or until jam thickened.
5. Pour into the container and store it in the fridge.

NUTRITION: Calories 16 Fat 0 g Carbohydrates 3.7 g Sugar 3.4 g Protein 0.1 g Cholesterol 0 mg

479. Warm Peach Compote

Preparation Time: 10 minutes

Cooking Time: 1 minute

Servings: 4

INGREDIENTS

- 4 peaches, peeled and chopped
- 1 tbsp water
- 1/2 tbsp cornstarch
- 1 tsp vanilla

DIRECTIONS

1. Add water, vanilla, and peaches into the instant pot.
2. Seal pot with lid and cook on high for 1 minute.
3. Once done, allow to release pressure naturally. Remove lid.
4. In a small bowl, whisk together 1 tablespoon of water and cornstarch and pour into the pot and stir well.
5. Serve and enjoy.

NUTRITION: Calories 66 Fat 0.4 g Carbohydrates 15 g Sugar 14.1 g Protein 1.4 g Cholesterol 0 mg

480. Spiced Pear Sauce

Preparation Time: 10 minutes

Cooking Time: 6 hours

Servings: 12

INGREDIENTS

- 8 pears, cored and diced
- 1/2 tsp ground cinnamon
- 1/4 tsp ground nutmeg
- 1/4 tsp ground cardamom
- 1 cup of water

DIRECTIONS

1. Add all ingredients into the instant pot and stir well.
2. Seal the pot with a lid and select slow cook mode and cook on low for 6 hours.
3. Mash the sauce using potato masher.
4. Pour into the container and store it in the fridge.

NUTRITION: Calories 81 Fat 0.2 g Carbohydrates 21.4 g Sugar 13.6 g Protein 0.5 g Cholesterol 0 mg

481. Honey Fruit Compote

Preparation Time: 10 minutes

Cooking Time: 3 minutes

Servings: 4

INGREDIENTS

- 1/3 cup honey
- 1 1/2 cups blueberries
- 1 1/2 cups raspberries

DIRECTIONS

1. Add all ingredients into the instant pot and stir well.
2. Seal pot with lid and cook on high for 3 minutes.
3. Once done, allow to release pressure naturally. Remove lid.
4. Serve and enjoy.

NUTRITION: Calories 141 Fat 0.5 g Carbohydrates 36.7 g Sugar 30.6 g Protein 1 g Cholesterol 0 mg

482. Creamy Brown Rice Pudding

Preparation Time: 10 minutes

Cooking Time: 20 minutes

Servings: 8

INGREDIENTS

- 1 cup of rice

- 1 cup of brown rice
- 1 cup of water
- 1 cup half and half
- 1/2 cup pecans, chopped
- 2 tsp vanilla
- 1 tbsp coconut butter
- 1/2 cup heavy cream
- Pinch of salt

DIRECTIONS

1. Add coconut butter into the instant pot and set the pot on sauté mode.
2. Add pecans into the pot and stir until toasted.
3. Add remaining ingredients except for heavy cream and vanilla. Stir well.
4. Seal pot with lid and cook on high for 20 minutes.
5. Once done, allow to release pressure naturally for 10 minutes then release remaining using quick release. Remove lid.
6. Add vanilla and heavy cream. Stir well and serve.

NUTRITION: Calories 276 Fat 10.9 g Carbohydrates 39.2 g Sugar 0.5 g Protein 5 g Cholesterol 21 mg

483. Lemon Cranberry Sauce

Preparation Time: 10 minutes

Cooking Time: 14 minutes

Servings: 8

INGREDIENTS

- 10 oz fresh cranberries
- 3/4 cup Swerve
- 1/4 cup water
- 1 tsp lemon zest

- 1 tsp vanilla extract

DIRECTIONS

1. Add cranberries and water into the instant pot.
2. Seal pot with lid and cook on high for 1 minute.
3. Once done, allow to release pressure naturally for 10 minutes then release remaining using quick release. Remove lid.
4. Set pot on sauté mode.
5. Add remaining ingredients and cook for 2-3 minutes.
6. Pour in container and store in fridge.

NUTRITION: Calories 21 Fat 0 g Carbohydrates 25.8 g Sugar 23.9 g Protein 0 g Cholesterol 0 mg

484. Blackberry Jam

Preparation Time: 10 minutes

Cooking Time: 6 hours

Servings: 6

INGREDIENTS

- 3 cups fresh blackberries
- 1/4 cup chia seeds
- 4 tbsp Swerve
- 1/4 cup fresh lemon juice
- 1/4 cup coconut butter

DIRECTIONS

1. Add all ingredients into the instant pot and stir well.
2. Seal the pot with a lid and select slow cook mode and cook on low for 6 hours.

3. Pour in container and store in fridge.

NUTRITION: Calories 101 Fat 6.8 g Carbohydrates 20 g Sugar 14.4 g Protein 2 g Cholesterol 0 mg

485. Chunky Apple Sauce

Preparation Time: 10 minutes

Cooking Time: 12 minutes

Servings: 16

INGREDIENTS

- 4 apples, peeled, cored and diced
- 1 tsp vanilla
- 4 pears, diced
- 2 tbsp cinnamon
- 1/4 cup maple syrup
- 3/4 cup water

DIRECTIONS

1. Add all ingredients into the instant pot and stir well.
2. Seal pot with lid and cook on high for 12 minutes.
3. Once done, allow to release pressure naturally for 10 minutes then release remaining using quick release. Remove lid.
4. Serve and enjoy.

NUTRITION: Calories 75 Fat 0.2 g Carbohydrates 19.7 g Sugar 13.9 g Protein 0.4 g Cholesterol 0 mg

486. Maple Syrup Cranberry Sauce

Preparation Time: 10 minutes

Cooking Time: 5 minutes

Servings: 8

INGREDIENTS

- 12 oz fresh cranberries, rinsed
- 1 apple, peeled, cored, and chopped
- 1/2 cup maple syrup
- 1/2 cup apple cider
- 1 tsp orange zest, grated
- 1 orange juice

DIRECTIONS

1. Add all ingredients into the instant pot and stir well.
2. Seal pot with lid and cook on high for 5 minutes.
3. Once done, allow to release pressure naturally for 10 minutes then release remaining using quick release. Remove lid.
4. Pour in container and store in fridge.

NUTRITION: Calories 101 Fat 0.1 g Carbohydrates 23.9 g Sugar 18.8 g Protein 0.2 g Cholesterol 0 mg

487. **Raisin Pecan Baked Apples**

Preparation Time: 10 minutes

Cooking Time: 4 minutes

Servings: 6

INGREDIENTS

- 6 apples, cored and cut into wedges
- 1 cup red wine
- 1/4 cup pecans, chopped
- 1/4 cup raisins
- 1/4 tsp nutmeg

- 1 tsp cinnamon
- 1/3 cup honey

DIRECTIONS

1. Add all ingredients into the instant pot and stir well.
2. Seal pot with lid and cook on high for 4 minutes.
3. Once done, allow to release pressure naturally for 10 minutes then release remaining using quick release. Remove lid.
4. Stir well and serve.

NUTRITION: Calories 229 Fat 0.9 g Carbohydrates 52.6 g Sugar 42.6 g Protein 1 g Cholesterol 0 mg

488. **Healthy Zucchini Pudding**

Preparation Time: 10 minutes

Cooking Time: 10 minutes

Servings: 4

INGREDIENTS

- 2 cups zucchini, shredded
- 1/4 tsp cardamom powder
- 5 oz half and half
- 5 oz almond milk
- 1/4 cup Swerve

DIRECTIONS

1. Add all ingredients except cardamom into the instant pot and stir well.
2. Seal pot with lid and cook on high for 10 minutes.
3. Once done, allow to release pressure naturally for 10 minutes then release

remaining using quick release. Remove lid.

4. Stir in cardamom and serve.

NUTRITION: Calories 137 Fat 12.6 g Carbohydrates 20.5 g Sugar 17.2 g Protein 2.6 g Cholesterol 13 mg

489. Cinnamon Apple Rice Pudding

Preparation Time: 10 minutes

Cooking Time: 15 minutes

Servings: 8

INGREDIENTS

- 1 cup of rice
- 1 tsp vanilla
- 1/4 apple, peeled and chopped
- 1/2 cup water
- 1 1/2 cup almond milk
- 1 tsp cinnamon
- 1 cinnamon stick

DIRECTIONS

1. Add all ingredients into the instant pot and stir well.
2. Seal pot with lid and cook on high for 15 minutes.
3. Once done, release pressure using quick release. Remove lid.
4. Stir and serve.

NUTRITION: Calories 206 Fat 11.5 g Carbohydrates 23.7 g Sugar 2.7 g Protein 3 g Cholesterol 0 mg

490. Coconut Risotto Pudding

Preparation Time: 10 minutes

Cooking Time: 20 minutes

Servings: 6

INGREDIENTS

- 3/4 cup rice
- 1/2 cup shredded coconut
- 1 tsp lemon juice
- 1/2 tsp vanilla
  - oz can coconut milk
- 1/4 cup maple syrup
- 1 1/2 cups water

DIRECTIONS

1. Add all ingredients into the instant pot and stir well.
2. Seal pot with lid and cook on high for 20 minutes.
3. Once done, allow to release pressure naturally for 10 minutes then release remaining using quick release. Remove lid.
4. Blend pudding mixture using an immersion blender until smooth.
5. Serve and enjoy.

NUTRITION: Calories 205 Fat 8.6 g Carbohydrates 29.1 g Sugar 9 g Protein 2.6 g Cholesterol 0 mg

491. Mediterranean Baked Apples

Servings: 4,

Cooking Time: 25 minutes

INGREDIENTS

- 1.5 pounds apples, peeled and sliced
- Juice from ½ lemon
- A dash of cinnamon

DIRECTIONS

1. Preheat the oven to 2500F.
2. Line a baking sheet with parchment paper then set aside.
3. In a medium bowl, apples with lemon juice and cinnamon.
4. Place the apples on the parchment paper-lined baking sheet.
5. Bake for 25 minutes until crisp.

NUTRITION:Calories: 90; Carbs: 23.9g; Protein: 0.5g; Fat: 0.3g

492. Mediterranean Diet Cookie Recipe

Servings: 12,

Cooking Time: 40 minutes

INGREDIENTS

- 1 tsp vanilla extract
- ½ tsp salt
- 4 large egg whites
- 1 ¼ cups sugar
- 2 cups toasted and skinned hazelnuts

DIRECTIONS

1. Preheat oven to 325oF and position oven rack in the center. Then line with baking paper your baking pan.
2. In a food processor, finely grind the hazelnuts and then transfer into a medium sized bowl.
3. In a large mixing bowl, on high speed beat salt and egg whites until stiff and there is formation of peaks. Then gently fold in the ground nut and vanilla until thoroughly mixed.
4. Drop a spoonful of the mixture onto prepared pan and bake the cookies for

twenty minutes or until lightly browned per batch. Bake 6 cookies per cookie sheet.

5. Let it cool on pan for five minutes before removing.

NUTRITION: Calorie per Servings: 173; Carbs: 23.0g; Protein: 3.1g; Fats: 7.6g

493. Mediterranean Style Fruit Medley

Servings: 7,

Cooking Time: 5 minutes

INGREDIENTS

- 4 fuyu persimmons, sliced into wedges
- 1 ½ cups grapes, halved
- 8 mint leaves, chopped
- 1 tablespoon lemon juice
- 1 tablespoon honey
- ½ cups almond, toasted and chopped

DIRECTIONS

1. Combine all Ingredients in a bowl.
2. Toss then chill before serving.

NUTRITION: Calories per serving:159; Carbs: 32g; Protein: 3g; Fat: 4g

494. Mediterranean Watermelon Salad

Servings: 6,

Cooking Time: 2 minutes

INGREDIENTS

- 6 cups mixed salad greens, torn

- 3 cups watermelon, seeded and cubed
- ½ cup onion, sliced
- 1 tablespoon extra-virgin olive oil
- 1/3 cup feta cheese, crumbled
- Cracked black pepper

DIRECTIONS

1. In a large bowl, mix all ingredients.
2. Toss to combine everything.
3. Allow to chill before serving.

NUTRITION: Calories: 91; Carbs: 15.2g; Protein: 1.9g; Fat: 2.8g

495. Melon Cucumber Smoothie

Servings: 2,

Cooking Time: 5 minutes

INGREDIENTS

- ½ cucumber
- 2 slices of melon
- 2 tablespoons lemon juice
- 1 pear, peeled and sliced
- 3 fresh mint leaves
- ½ cup almond milk

DIRECTIONS

1. Place all Ingredients in a blender.
2. Blend until smooth.
3. Pour in a glass container and allow to chill in the fridge for at least 30 minutes.

NUTRITION: Calories: 253; Carbs: 59.3g; Protein: 5.7g; Fat: 2.1g

496. Peanut Banana Yogurt Bowl

Servings: 4,

Cooking Time: 15 minutes

INGREDIENTS

- 4 cups Greek yogurt
- 2 medium bananas, sliced
- ¼ cup creamy natural peanut butter
- ¼ cup flax seed meal
- 1 teaspoon nutmeg

DIRECTIONS

1. Divide the yogurt between four bowls and top with banana, peanut butter, and flax seed meal.
2. Garnish with nutmeg.
3. Chill before serving.

NUTRITION: Calories: 370; Carbs: 47.7g; Protein: 22.7g; Fat: 10.6g

497. Pomegranate and Lychee Sorbet

Servings: 6,

Cooking Time: 5 minutes

INGREDIENTS

- ¾ cup dragon fruit cubes
- 8 lychees, peeled and pitted
- Juice from 1 lemon
- 3 tablespoons stevia sugar
- 2 tablespoons pomegranate seeds

DIRECTIONS

1. In a blender, combine, the dragon fruit, lychees, lemon, and stevia sugar.

2. Pulse until smooth.
3. Pour the mixture in a container with lid and place inside the fridge.
4. Allow sorbet to harden for at least 8 hours.
5. Sprinkle with pomegranate seeds before serving.

NUTRITION: Calories per serving:214; Carbs: 30.4g; Protein: 1.9g; Fat: 1.2g

498. Pomegranate Granita with Lychee

Servings: 7,

Cooking Time: 5 minutes

INGREDIENTS

- 500 millimeters pomegranate juice, organic and sugar-free
- 1 cup water
- ½ cup lychee syrup
- 2 tablespoons lemon juice
- 4 mint leaves
- 1 cup fresh lychees, pitted and sliced

DIRECTIONS

1. Place all Ingredients in a large pitcher.
2. Place inside the fridge to cool before serving.

NUTRITION:Calories: 96; Carbs: 23.8g; Protein: 0.4g; Fat: 0.4g

499. Roasted Berry and Honey Yogurt Pops

Servings: 8,

Cooking Time: 15 minutes

INGREDIENTS

- 12 ounces mixed berries
- A dash of sea salt
- 2 tablespoons honey
- 2 cups whole Greek yogurt
- ½ small lemon, juice

DIRECTIONS

1. Preheat the oven to 3500F.
2. Line a baking sheet with parchment paper then set aside.
3. In a medium bowl, toss the berries with sea salt and honey.
4. Pour the berries on the prepared baking sheet.
5. Roast for 30 minutes while stirring halfway.
6. While the fruit is roasting, blend the Greek yogurt and lemon juice. Add honey to taste if desired.
7. Once the berries are done, cool for at least ten minutes.
8. Fold the berries into the yogurt mixture.
9. Pour into popsicle molds and allow to freeze for at least 8 hours.
10. Serve chilled.

NUTRITION:Calories: 177; Carbs: 24.8g; Protein: 3.2g; Fat: 7.9g

500. Scrumptious Cake with Cinnamon

Servings: 8,

Cooking Time: 40 minutes

INGREDIENTS

- 1 lemon
- 4 eggs

- 1 tsp cinnamon
- ¼ lb. sugar
- ½ lb. ground almonds

DIRECTIONS

1. Preheat oven to 350oF. Then grease a cake pan and set aside.
2. On high speed, beat for three minutes the sugar and eggs or until the volume is doubled.
3. Then with a spatula, gently fold in the lemon zest, cinnamon and almond flour until well mixed.
4. Then pour batter on prepared pan and bake for forty minutes or until golden brown.
5. Let cool before serving.

NUTRITION: Calorie per Servings: 253; Carbs: 21.1g; Protein: 8.8g; Fats: 16.3g

501. **Smoothie Bowl with Dragon Fruit**

Servings: 4,

Cooking Time: 5 minutes

INGREDIENTS

- ¼ of dragon fruit, peeled and sliced
- 1 cup frozen berries
- 2 cups baby greens (mixed)
- ½ cup coconut meat

DIRECTIONS

1. Place all Ingredients in a blender and pulse until smooth.
2. Place on a bowl and allow to cool in the fridge for at least 20 minutes.
3. Garnish with whatever fruits or nuts available in your fridge.

NUTRITION: Calories: 190; Carbs: 19g; Protein: 5g; Fat: 13g

502. **Soothing Red Smoothie**

Servings: 2,

Cooking Time: 3 minutes

INGREDIENTS

- 4 plums, pitted
- ¼ cup raspberry
- ¼ cup blueberry
- 1 tablespoon lemon juice
- 1 tablespoon linseed oil

DIRECTIONS

1. Place all Ingredients in a blender.
2. Blend until smooth.
3. Pour in a glass container and allow to chill in the fridge for at least 30 minutes.

NUTRITION: Calories: 201; Carbs: 36.4g; Protein: 0.8g; Fat: 7.1g

503. **Strawberry and Avocado Medley**

Servings: 4,
Cooking Time: 5 minutes

INGREDIENTS

- 2 cups strawberry, halved
- 1 avocado, pitted and sliced
- 2 tablespoons slivered almonds

DIRECTIONS

1. Place all Ingredients in a mixing bowl.
2. Toss to combine.

3. Allow to chill in the fridge before serving.

NUTRITION: Calories**: 107; Carbs: 9.9g; Protein: 1.6g; Fat: 7.8g

504. **Strawberry Banana Greek Yogurt Parfaits**

Servings: 4,
Cooking Time: 5 minutes

INGREDIENTS

- 1 cup plain Greek yogurt, chilled
- 1 cup pepitas
- ½ cup chopped strawberries
- ½ banana, sliced

DIRECTIONS

1. In a parfait glass, add the yogurt at the bottom of the glass.
2. Add a layer of pepitas, strawberries, and bananas.
3. Continue to layer the Ingredients until the entire glass is filled.

NUTRITION: Calories per serving:387; Carbs: 69.6g; Protein: 18.1g; Fat: 1g

505. **Summertime Fruit Salad**

Servings: 6,
Cooking Time: 5 minutes

INGREDIENTS

- 1-pound strawberries, hulled and sliced thinly
- 3 medium peaches, sliced thinly

- 6 ounces blueberries
- 1 tablespoon fresh mint, chopped
- 2 tablespoons lemon juice
- 1 tablespoon honey
- 2 teaspoons balsamic vinegar

DIRECTIONS

1. In a salad bowl, combine all ingredients.
2. Gently toss to coat all ingredients.
3. Chill for at least 30 minutes before serving.

NUTRITION: Calories**: 146; Carbs: 22.8g; Protein: 8.1g; Fat: 3.4g

506. **Sweet Tropical Medley Smoothie**

Servings: 4, Preparation Time: 10 minutes
Cooking time: 5 minutes

INGREDIENTS

- 1 banana, peeled
- 1 sliced mango
- 1 cup fresh pineapple
- ½ cup coconut water

DIRECTIONS

1. Place all Ingredients in a blender.
2. Blend until smooth.
3. Pour in a glass container and allow to chill in the fridge for at least 30 minutes.

NUTRITION: Calories per serving:73 ; Carbs: 18.6g; Protein: 0.8g; Fat: 0.5g.

CONCLUSION

The Mediterranean diet is the regime you've been waiting for that won't break your bank, isolate you from your friends and family, or cause you to bounce back to a size seventeen after only a few months. By now, you should have a keen understanding of what eating like the Mediterranean's means - and if you weren't entirely won over by the promise of carbs for life, we hope the weight loss and health benefits alone have swayed you in the direction of changing your life. When you commit to a Mediterranean diet, you commit to lots of healthy fats and oils, lots of time with your friends and family, and lots more years of health to come in the future. Don't give up, and don't forget that your body is yours, and yours only – so treat it kindly! Thanks for sticking with us as we walked you through all the ins and outs of the Mediterranean diet, and we wish you the best of luck on your journey towards a healthier, thinner, and more coastal-minded you

Food Avoid   White Sugar

French Fries 450 CAL   Bagels 350 CAL

Red Meat   Muffins

* Whip Cream   * Can Soup

peanut Butter   White Bread

Fruit Juice   Resturant Desserts

* Ice Cream   Drive Thru FAST Food

* Crakers   Butter

* Cream Cheese

Jam preserves

MAYO Ba.

* Coffee Cream

* Onion Rings

Lg Coffee Drinks

* pie

* pancakes, Butter & Syrup

Grondnola

* Bottle Tea

* pizza

soy Bean Oil

* Burger 300 cal

* cookies pretzel

Printed in the USA
CPSIA information can be obtained
at www.ICGtesting.com
LVHW071308010224
770626LV00011B/610